Never Say Die

A DOCTOR AND PATIENT TALK ABOUT BREAST CANCER

D1072145

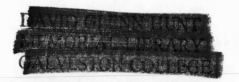

DAVID GLENN HUNT
MEMORIAL LIBRARY
GALVESTON COLLEGE

Never Say Die

A DOCTOR AND PATIENT TALK ABOUT BREAST CANCER

Lucy Shapero
Anthony A. Goodman,
M.D., F.A.C.S.

*Clinical Assistant Professor of Surgery
The University of Miami School of Medicine;
Private surgical practice*

Foreword by
Alfred S. Ketcham, M.D.

*Former Clinical Director and
Chief of the Surgical Branch of
The National Cancer Institute*

APPLETON-CENTURY-CROFTS/New York

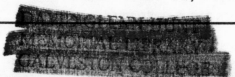

NOTICE: The authors and publisher of this book have, as far as it is possible to do so, taken care to make certain that recommendations regarding treatment and use of drugs are correct and compatible with the standards generally accepted at the time of publication. However, knowledge in medical science is constantly changing. As new information becomes available, changes in treatment and in the use of drugs may become necessary. The reader is urged to consult her physician for professional advice in dealing with any serious or potentially serious medical problem.

Copyright © 1980 by Lucy Shapero and Anthony A. Goodman

All rights reserved. This book, or any parts thereof, may not be used or reproduced in any manner without written permission. For information, address Appleton-Century-Crofts, 292 Madison Avenue, New York, N.Y. 10017.

80 81 82 83 84 / 10 9 8 7 6 5 4 3 2 1

Prentice-Hall International, Inc., *London*
Prentice-Hall of Australia, Pty. Ltd., *Sydney*
Prentice-Hall of India Private Limited, *New Delhi*
Prentice-Hall of Japan, Inc., *Tokyo*
Prentice-Hall of Southeast Asia (Pte.) Ltd., *Singapore*
Whitehall Books Ltd., *Wellington, New Zealand*

Library of Congress Cataloging in Publication Data

Shapero, Lucy, 1932–
    Never say die.

    Includes index.
    1. Breast—Cancer. 2. Breast—Cancer—United States—Biography.
3. Shapero, Lucy, 1932–   I. Goodman, Anthony A., joint author.
II. Title. [DNLM: 1. Breast neoplasms—Popular works. WP870 S529n]
RC280.B8S49   616.99'449   80-17944
ISBN 0-8385-6718-5

Text design: Judith F. Warm
Cover design: RD Graphics

PRINTED IN THE UNITED STATES OF AMERICA

To Jack
L. S.

To Katie — always my snug harbor
A. A. G.

Contents

Foreword

The privilege of a cancer patient, Lucy Shapero, to tell her personal story with its message and moral is uniquely dramatized in NEVER SAY DIE. Similarly, the surgeon, Anthony Goodman, interweaves his philosophy and technical facts and experience with Lucy's story in such an appealing way that NEVER SAY DIE is read with anticipation and excitement. We hear Lucy's plea for recognition as an individual who wants to know about her condition and participate in her treatment planning. And Tony asks for understanding and reason in dealing with his recommendations, decisions, and actions. Together they create an important and powerful partnership.

The surgeon's primary obligation is to offer the patient the treatment which combines the best opportunity for cure while still offering a reasonable and acceptable quality of survival. All patients should be encouraged to seek a second opinion from an experienced, reliable physician interested in the treatment of the cancer patient. Whatever treatment is decided on can then be undertaken with optimism both by the doctor and the patient, having discussed available options and probable outcomes.

Breast cancer is not necessarily the same disease in each patient and its growth characteristics can be most variable from one patient to another. Therefore, the same treatment is not necessarily best for each patient.

Each woman must be offered the opportunity to participate in the decision as to what her course of treatment will be, but she must educate herself in every way possible in order to understand and communicate with her physician at this crucial time. Ultimately, she must be able to trust her personal physician and rely on his recommendations.

The art and science of surgery and oncology are constantly

being developed and expanded. As Tony indicates in his portions, perhaps time will show us that removal of only the tumor mass itself and leaving the apparently normal breast tissue (lumpectomy) will result in the same cure rates as for the more radical procedures. Regular follow-ups and further laboratory studies must be part of the continuing treatment plan. In the early stages of cancer growth, proper treatment may afford an almost 100 percent cure. However, a cancer patient who has been treated and is "cured," like Lucy, must be diligently alert to the signs and symptoms of possible cancer recurrence or the development of a new unrelated cancer. Such awareness and self-monitoring must not interfere with a normal productive lifestyle. Recurrent new cancers can often be treated with very convincing and favorable cure rates. Lucy's experience is testimony to this.

Cancer of the breast is the number one killer of women between the ages of 35 and 60. Yet it need not be such a frequent killer if women could be convinced that it is an illness that is curable if recognized early. Cancer is best faced by honesty to oneself and to those who will offer support during the periods of expected and normally reactive depressions. Open and honest discussions about the cancer problem are most helpful, not only for the patient, but for her family as well.

Looking ahead to a normal life while being treated for cancer is only part of the expected success in facing and living with the cancer crisis. There must be a satisfying quality of life associated with survival. It is pleasing to return the patient to her home and family and community through aggressive physical rehabilitation, but the cosmetic and emotional restoration of the patient is of equal importance. With present techniques of plastic surgery and more acceptable prosthetic aids, all women can be afforded a breast that is cosmetically acceptable in most situations.

The patient who looks ahead to the future realizing that early breast cancer growths are totally removable and highly curable will be that patient who is most often cured. In those instances where treatment fails in the first attack, there are several other approaches to treatment which can be concurrently or repetitively instituted. Cancer can be controlled and even be cured. If we can develop this optimism in patients and physicians, then the present dilemma of fear and delay in recognition will be largely eliminated. Lucy and Tony offer hope and education to all breast cancer patients, their families, and their physicians.

Alfred S. Ketcham, M.D.

Professor of Surgery
Chief, Division of Surgical Oncology
University of Miami School of Medicine, Miami, Florida
Former Clinical Director and Chief of the Surgical Branch
of the National Cancer Institute, Bethesda, Maryland

Preface

Until now, most books about breast cancer, written for the lay public, have been written by women who are within months of having their mastectomies. The pages are still wet with their tears. They battle the emotions of sorrow and fear, anger and loss of sexuality.

Our book is written from a different perspective, or rather from two different perspectives. Lucy was diagnosed as having breast cancer ten years ago and has lived through the initial treatment and recovery, a metastasis, and more treatment and recovery. Tony is a surgeon who treats many cases of breast cancer each year and is, not incidentally, related to Lucy.

We have written the book in two parallel strands — Lucy's experiences as a patient; Tony's as a surgeon.

We have been disturbed by the misinformation disseminated by newspapers, television, and magazines. The very nature of media is to sensationalize, while the evolution of breast cancer treatment has been measured in millimeters, not miles; conveyed in whispers, not shouted in headlines.

Perspective demands that we examine the most important aspect of having breast cancer: the divergent concepts of living with or dying from the disease. Breast cancer patients, unlike patients with other types of cancer, will live under the Sword of Damocles for five, ten, even twenty years.

We have lived through ten of those years — experiencing fear and joy, pain and frustration, metastasis and remission. The perspective of time is one we hope to share with our readers.

The treatment of breast cancer is changing. Because the science of medicine is fluid, what was considered a fad ten years ago is viewed today as serious and legitimate.

In many ways, patients have forced doctors to reexamine their research. No longer satisfied with dogma, the lay public demands exploration and reevaluation of ideas.

If doctors are willing to reshape their thinking, patients, too, must become more informed. They must do their homework. As options open and choices appear, they must be aware of what alternatives they have. Patients are consumers, and they must learn to shop for the proper medical treatment.

Breast cancer is a sweeping, perplexing, personal experience. Yet the patient does not exist in a vacuum. She, her doctors, family, and friends share her illness. While there may be historical similarities, the disease varies in each person and her support group must be aware of the similarities and differences.

The subject of breast cancer should be viewed from the perspective of the patient and her doctor, recognizing that the ultimate goals of both should be identical. The doctor must realize that an educated patient will be more helpful in her own treatment. The patient must accept the responsibility of participating in medical as well as personal decisions. Cooperations of this kind can only be based on honesty.

We approach our material from two viewpoints: the patient's and the doctor's, the personal and the clinical. Both are essential in order to understand the complex properties of the disease. Both demand attention for the purposes of education, attitude, and perspective.

These two points of view symbolize what we feel is most important when dealing with breast cancer. Honest, open, respectful communication is a requisite for positive relationships. Living with cancer depends on the will and affirmation those kinds of relationships inspire.

Acknowledgments

To Doreen Berne, who prodded, taught, and exceeded the role of editor by being my friend; to Ralph Scott, who listened and cared; and to all of my friends, unnamed here, whose support and love have sustained me: thank you.

L. S.

My deepest thanks to my close friend and associate, Dr. Arthur I. Segaul, for his support, teachings, and his readiness to adopt new methods for our patients as time and experience dictated; to Dr. Paul Freiberg for the care he has taken in the chemotherapy of our patients and his advice in the preparation of the chapter on chemotherapy in this book; to Dr. James Collins, who has brought the expertise in radiation therapy to our community that allowed us to take the step to lumpectomy and radiation in the treatment of breast cancer, and for his advice in the preparation of this book; to Katherine Anne Goodman for her invaluable assistance in the preparation of the glossary; to Jan Foy for painful hours of deciphering my dictation and handwriting.

And deepest appreciation to Doreen Berne, editor and friend, for her continuous encouragement from before the start to the finish of this book, and to Kate Brown of Appleton-Century-Crofts for her gentle persuasion.

A. A. G.

Never Say Die

A DOCTOR AND
PATIENT TALK ABOUT
BREAST CANCER

1

In the Beginning

Lucy

At a party, a woman who had breast cancer approached me and asked how I was faring with this book. She added, strongly, "I hope you present my point of view—that I don't want to know anything. I don't want to make any decisions. I just want to be put to sleep and have done what needs to be done." She smiled as she spoke, but I knew that she was serious. So I responded that every book must have a point of view and this one would reflect mine. I suggested she write one for herself.

And I do recognize that my experiences and feelings won't be shared by everyone. Learning to live with cancer has taken time. Happily, I have had the time. I have had time to make mistakes and learn from those mistakes. I have had time to analyze prejudices and change priorities. I have had time to explore relationships and contemplate philosophies. And I have changed. Though I still have metastasic cancer, I have gained a sensibility I didn't have before I got sick.

Ten years ago, when I learned I had breast cancer, I was certain I was going to die. I was only thirty-seven years old, but I planned no further. For me, cancer was a single disease marked by terrible pain and a slow, torturous death. What interest I had was based on fear. I was medically ignorant. I simply allowed what happened to happen. If I had admitted that the disease was a possibility in my life (there is a high incidence of breast cancer in my family) and had learned about the treatment procedures before I was diagnosed, I could have made the decisions then that I live with today. But I didn't want to deal with the unpleasantness. The thought of breast cancer was ugly. So why think of it?

The surgeon I chose to perform the mastectomy was highly regarded in the medical community. I placed myself in his hands. I had always considered myself a thinking person.

1

Never one to trust others' attitudes and opinions, I had questioned, probed, discussed, and read for myself. I had always loved a good argument. However, with my own disease, fear overcame my independence. The problems I faced were so laden with catastrophe that I turned away. I asked no questions. When I realized later that I would live rather than die with cancer, I began to educate myself.

For the layman, doctors are the best source of information. But doctors dislike questioners. I have asked many doctors what they tell their patients. Do they tell them the whole truth? Do they answer real *and* implied questions? Doctors reply, invariably, that they try to be candid and reassuring but that they also try to avoid frightening details. They feel we might not comprehend the difficult implications of medical terminology. They worry that we might become irrational if told the facts and possibilities of a serious illness. But they agree that trust is a most important factor in the doctor/patient relationship. However, one important element is often omitted in establishing that relationship. That element is time. I realize that doctors are educated, well-trained professionals who are busy with the business of keeping people alive. I know too that their concern for the quality of life can be diminished by the quantities of lives they see. How much better it would be for doctor and patient both if they could spend more time together—time for the doctor to determine how much truth a patient might want and be able to understand; time for the patient to demonstrate her ability to comprehend, to learn her options so that she might plan her course of action intelligently. It is far easier for a doctor to treat a patient and walk away than to be deterred by queries and discuss alternatives.

I needed to know what my disease was. I wanted an idea of what I could expect. So I read. I read medical texts. I read first-person accounts. I read philosophy. I read psychology. And luckily, I was able to talk to Tony about what I read and how it applied to me. Because he is related to me, and because he is a surgeon, he had access to my doctors and to my records and could talk to me about the specifics of my case rather than relating only statistical generalities.

Knowledge is the most important tool I have in dealing with cancer. It enables me to make educated decisions about how I will live. And living is what this book is about. But it is about more than just living with cancer. It is about living with myself, my husband, my children, my family, and my friends.

Every woman who has breast cancer is a survivor with a story to tell. My story has the added adventure of elapsed time. And time is what makes it special. So much of what we read deals with cancer death. I write of life.

Tony

In January, 1970, while Lucy was preparing for her breast biopsy, I was a senior surgical resident on one of the Harvard teaching services in Boston. As with most of my colleagues at that level of training, I was very confident of my surgical judgment and knowledge, and had a hefty ego regarding my technical skill in the operating room. At that stage most of us felt that there were only a few fine points left to be learned as we approached our year as chief resident. By then we had finished almost six years of postgraduate training, had hundreds of surgical cases under our belts, and felt that the supervision provided by our senior attending staff was unnecessary and, in many cases, confining. We labored under the misconception that by the time we finished our year as "chiefs" there would be little more for us to learn and little room for technical improvement in our operative skills. In the operating room we viewed the operative prowess of most of the surgeons with an unyieldingly critical eye, and through the "retrospectoscope" came down hard on any less than perfect result. The surgeons' good results were viewed as having occurred despite, rather than because of, surgical skill.

There are in every training program a handful of "heroes" —men who shine primarily because of their incredible operative skill, usually the result of an enormous case load experience. As much as the lesser surgeons are scorned by the residents, the "heroes" are praised and emulated. As senior residents and chief residents, we tended to be very blind to the weaknesses and gaps in our knowledge and skills. We were all counting the days until we would be on our own, performing as our idols performed for us.

JUST A GENERAL SURGEON

General surgeons suffer a strong ego blow at the hands of the public. Our field is generally relegated to the realm of the nonspecialist. We still stiffen when asked if we are specialists or "just" general surgeons. In fact, the large number of diseases still treated by the general surgeon makes general surgery one of the more difficult and demanding fields in which to stay current. Indeed, in the case of the patient with multiple systems injuries or problems which involve many surgical specialties, the general surgeon assumes control, directs the patient's care, and assigns priorities and modes of treatment. I explain this not to praise the general surgeon, but to emphasize the fact that as a senior resident or chief resident, one has finished four to six years of training in a multiplicity of surgical specialties, including substantial experience in almost all of the surgical subspecialties (gynecology, orthopedics, cardiovascular surgery, neurosurgery, plastic surgery). From that lofty self-image, the new surgeon experiences a long, plummeting fall when first confronted with a problem which points out a major gap in one's knowledge.

HALSTED'S LEGACY

Surgery of the breast has always been the undisputed domain of the general surgeon. In many other disease areas there are overlapping fields of interest among the specialties. The general surgeon competes for thyroid and parotid surgery with the head and neck surgeons, for esophageal surgery with the chest surgeon, and for adrenal surgery with the urologist. But the gynecologist rarely performs definitive breast biopsies or radical breast surgery, despite the fact that most breast "lumps" are brought to the gynecologist's attention first. The reason for this probably stems from the history of surgery of the breast, which only really came into its own under the famous William Halsted of Johns Hopkins. Halsted was a general surgeon who, besides being the father of the residency system of surgical training in this country, was also the major innovator of radical surgery for breast cancer. Even today, this tradition remains unchallenged, and surgery of the breast is undeniably under the aegis of the general surgeon.

In January, 1970, a phone call from my sister-in-law, Betty, all but crumpled years of ego building and confidence in my own judgment and expertise. Betty had called to tell me that her sister, Lucy, then age 37, was going into the hospital for a breast biopsy and possible mastectomy. She asked me a long series of questions regarding technique, procedures, options, and prognosis. This was combined with the confusion that is so prevalent in a literate public bombarded by the partial truths of such "medical journals" as *Reader's Digest* and *Time* magazine. But suddenly I was at a total loss to advise her. All the hours I had spent with anxious patients and families awaiting breast biopsies evaporated, and I was terrified that I might give wrong or outdated advice to someone I loved.

The face of modern surgery changes with dizzying speed today, and even basic textbooks are years out of date at the time of publication. The surgical literature is overwhelming in volume and scope, and often contradictory papers appear within a few weeks of each other in the same journal. I was afraid my facts and statistics were going to be outdated or wrong. This had not bothered me before—I felt I could do my best on the basis of the facts as I knew them, gleaned from current teaching rounds and journals. But suddenly the involvement of someone dear to me made me unsure of my information. I no longer had what one of my own "heroes" used to refer to as the "valor of the noncombatant." I *was* a combatant, and I was terribly uncomfortable with the involvement.

This involvement led to a hurried search for facts, and the busy schedule I was keeping precluded any lengthy library searches of the surgical and oncological literature. So, since I was literally surrounded by the vast wealth of experience and knowledge of my professors and senior attending surgeons I began polling them for the facts I needed. Options regarding technique, prognosis, and follow-up treatment were first on the list. Then came the more difficult decisions regarding adjunctive versus delayed hormone manipulation, chemotherapy, and radiation. I gathered the information as best I could and was left with the overwhelming impression that the multiplicity of ideas, facts, and fantasies was going to make rational choices difficult for the doctors, and nearly impossible for Lucy and her family.

There were major decisions to be made, and both Lucy and I were at a disadvantage. Lucy's choices were made even more difficult because she did not know what questions to ask. I had not yet had the experience of treating patients with breast cancer and following them for a few years. And, unfortunately, Lucy and I did not communicate directly at that time. I relayed my data and suggestions through Betty.

In the last ten years, we have lived through the results of all those decisions. Lucy has endured much in the way of conflicting advice and doctors who were at cross purposes with her and with each other. She has been treated with surgery, radiation, hormone ablation, and more radiation. She has lived five years believing herself free of cancer, and five more years knowing her cancer had spread. However, Lucy Shapero is alive and well and living in Louisville. Now, ten years later, she is clinically free of disease, she understands her disease, and she lives with it. And now we talk directly — discuss, communicate, and help each other.

Much has been written on the subject of breast cancer, largely by women who have recently undergone mastectomy. These women seem very concerned with their cosmetic tragedy but have little or no concept of cure or recurrence, of living or dying. They have faced the threat of death from breast cancer, but have not yet dealt with the reality of living with it.

Lucy has experienced all of this, the good and the bad; doctors she could deal with, and those with whom she could not. We both hope this book will spell out in understandable terms exactly what breast cancer is, how we deal with it, and the many options open to the patient. At the same time we think reliving some of Lucy's feelings may prepare patients for living with their own feelings, and lessen their sense of isolation, confusion, and loss.

Today, most breast cancers can be controlled even when they cannot be cured. An understanding of the factors involved in deciding courses of treatment is vital to every breast cancer patient, because quality of life can be at least as important as the actual length of life.

The days should be over when a lone surgeon will assess the problem and present the patient with a fait accompli as to choice of treatment. Every woman who has or may have breast cancer has an obligation to educate herself well enough to be able to participate in the choices of treatment available to her.

It is our hope that a better understanding of the disease process, natural history, and choices of treatment will enable patients to participate actively in their own treatments and, to a large extent, exert personal control over their own destinies.

2

About Cancer

Lucy

If I could pick one moment in time to return to, it would be the moment when the Grand Tetons burst from the earth. I like to think it happened that way. One minute there were wide, endless plains. The next, the valley was split by a vomiting earth, casting up raw, awesome mountains—snow-covered, glacier-sided, rimmed at their base with glorious flowers. I would wake from my sleep—be awakened by the ground-trembling, boulder-splitting roar. And as I watched, aghast, the sun would rise, bathing the tips of the peaks in pink and orange. There could be no more beautiful sight.

Grand Tetons means, in French, "big tits." The men who named them must have considered that the ultimate compliment. It seems we have been a breast-worshiping society far longer than I had realized.

For my husband Jack and me, vacation is a time of renewal. We leave our world behind and step into another dimension. Away from home, there is time and space to think about home. Put our worries and nuisances into new perspective. Or forget about home. Rediscover the pleasure of talking to each other, not about business or children or money or no money. Talk about feelings and dreams and fears. Of course, there is always cancer. It never leaves us. But, on vacations, in the Tetons, we play make-believe. We push the real world into the background and live for right now. There is no yesterday. There is no tomorrow. Today, summer, 1979, the mountains are all.

Home again. And the dinner table conversation centers around the latest victim of cancer. "They cut her open and she was so filled with it they just sewed her back up again." "There's nothing to be done." "She has lung involvement but she's taking chemotherapy." "She's so brave." "It's so sad."

I go to my room and stand in front of the mirror. Objectively, my image stares back. Healthy. I look so healthy. And there is a sparkle, a joy, an expectancy mirrored there. Nine, five, even three years ago I didn't look this way. I didn't think this way. I certainly didn't feel this way.

"Am I crazy? Am I a fool? Am I still denying the truth?" I whisper the questions to my reflection. And I hear myself answer, "No. No. No. Celebrate. You are winning. The rounds in your fight aren't limited to ten or fifteen. It can go on and on as long as you can come to the center of the ring. And there is time. Use the time. Recognize it as a healer, a friend. It will restore your strength. It will heal your bruises. But know what you're fighting. Know its tactics. Know that between punches it is stalking, planning, waiting. Dancing, diverting, energizing."

I had given myself this speech yesterday and last week and for months and years before tonight. I believed it. I wanted to believe it. I needed to believe it, and I still need to believe it.

Nine years ago I hadn't even thought of it. Nine years ago I thought myself immortal. I was Lucy. Jack's wife. Mother of Ken, Rob, and Cathy. I had returned to Louisville after graduating from college. Before I went away, I had lived the life my parents had planned for me. And I had adapted. I did what everyone else did. I went where they went. I interested myself in their interests. But inside, there was turmoil. A secret me. Different. A me that flew deep into my books. I dreamed of being every character in every book I read. I rewrote them to better fit myself. I wasn't interested in the activities at school. I wasn't interested in playing hockey or singing in the glee club. Or being teacher's pet. Yet I never thought of rebelling. I hated confrontation. I wanted to conform. It was enough that I knew I was different.

College changed all that. At first I was frightened. Everyone seemed smart, articulate, confident. No one sat back and accepted anything. Teachers were questioned and doubted. Classmates were challenged by other students and by teachers. Authors were criticized, appraised, dissected. I was silent and unsure. Unsure of my judgment. Unsure of how I would be judged. And finally I ventured an opinion. People listened. I wrote a poem and offered it. It was critiqued and I was asked for more. And I began to trust. My differences were accepted. My differences were respected. Another opinion. A variant viewpoint. I revealed myself—and liked myself.

I came home and it was as if I had never been away. Except for the trust and approval I felt for the person I was. I had learned a lot.

When I married Jack, I wanted to be a good wife—whatever that was. Publicly, I took care of him. Privately, I took care of myself. I missed the camaraderie of college—the poetry readings, the string quartets, the drama workshops. But our marriage was good. And when I wasn't taking care of home and husband and children, I was reading and writing and dreaming. I still performed the expected ceremonies—holiday dinners, volunteer work, driving groups. But I was ambivalent about what I was doing. And I began to search for the elusive something that would make me feel important—that would make me be important.

Breast cancer had no part in my plans. Breast cancer was some other woman's misfortune—a forbidding thought, too horrible to dwell on.

My father died of cancer of the colon. When it was diagnosed, the doctors told him that he had from six months to a year to live. They meant six months. His death devastated me.

After he was operated on he came home. He grew strong. He could walk for miles. He went back to work—but he didn't work. He sat in his office until it was time to go home. My mother knew this and it worried her. She wanted him to use his time to live—to live until he died. She asked me to talk to him. It was a strange request to make of a daughter. I worried about it as I drove to meet with him. My father had invited me to lunch to celebrate my fifth wedding anniversary.

I sat across the desk from him. Without thinking any further I began, "Daddy, I know you have cancer and I know it's spread to your liver and the doctors say there's nothing to be done . . . but I love you so much. We have so much to share. Don't give up. Please don't give up now. There will be more good times. I know there will. We need you. I need you." We were in each other's arms. There were tears, smiles, soothings. We talked then — really talked. He admitted his hopelessness. The radiation treatment had depleted him. The second opinion he had sought in New York had discouraged him. He knew he was going to die. He knew how he would die. But he and I decided that afternoon that he wasn't dead yet. He could fight. He would live while he could.

I had felt so presumptuous. How could I be critical? How could I venture to know how he felt? But I needed him. I loved him. I couldn't bear to lose him.

I watched him die. He didn't have unbearable pain. He never gave up trying to live. He just got weaker and tireder. As he came closer to death, he became less interested — not in us, but in our problems. He felt he had done what he could and now was his time to rest.

I had never intimately experienced death until my father died. His was my first acquaintance with fatal cancer. My mother had had a disease called cystic mastitis and had both breasts removed when she was forty-one to prevent the possibility of her developing breast cancer. My aunt had had breast cancer and a resultant mastectomy when she was forty-five. Today both live healthy, active lives. My grandmother had breast cancer but she died, not from cancer, when I was two. I didn't know her.

When my mother was operated on, I remembered my father telling me that my mother's breasts had been removed. I was embarrassed. It was such a personal thing. A woman's private experience. And a personal problem between a man and his wife. Just to know made me feel as if I were prying. I was sixteen. My body had become very important to me. I couldn't imagine dealing with the loss of part of it — that part of it. How could my mother handle such gross mutilation? How could my father handle my mother's mutilation? She would be hideous. Would he find her so? Could he still love her? Could she allow his love? I watched them carefully. And I found no change in their relationship. My mother undressed in front of us. We couldn't help seeing her flattened chest. I tried to ignore her. I learned not to see. I never considered that if she had not had the mastectomies, breast cancer might have been her fate.

I disregarded the theory that the tendency toward breast cancer was inherited. I didn't want to think of it. It was too unpleasant and I was young and sure of my immortality. I seldom examined my breasts. Irrationally, I presumed that if I didn't check them, no lumps would occur. But I fantasized about being breastless — which is really what breast cancer meant to me — maimed, disfigured, ugly. The possibility became a fearful, recurring nightmare. I talked to Jack about it. I asked him if he could love me if I had no breasts. Unhesitatingly, he always answered yes, of course, don't worry. We both thought only of mutilation. We didn't think of death. Neither my mother nor my aunt nor my grandmother had died of breast cancer. They were just disfigured. My father had died, but his cancer had been a different kind. Nothing could happen to me.

But it did happen. And we have all changed. We have learned that losing a breast is, in itself, insignificant. Living is what is important. We have learned that each day might bring an unexpected joy and that suffering and sadness can result in growth and understanding. We have seen our family cope with despair and not be hideously scarred by it — rather, we have found a greater empathy and awareness of each other.

I have breast cancer. I think about it every day. But I am gloriously alive. And I celebrate my life.

Tony

DEFINING TERMS

For Lucy, a cancer meant deformity, pain, death, the loss of her father. For most people, the word *cancer* evokes a number of immediate gut reactions, but fear is the most universal. Hardly a day goes by without some mention of cancer, whether in magazines or on television or in connection with someone we know. Yet the real nature of cancer remains poorly defined and poorly understood by the general public. For one thing, cancer tends to be regarded as a single disease, when in fact it includes scores of different diseases with many different characteristics. The many types of cancers vary in their causative agents, populations of patients attacked, susceptibility to treatment, aggressiveness, and ultimate lethality or curability. Cancers may range from basal cell carcinomas of the skin, which are slow-growing, easily treated, and rarely kill anyone, to the anaplastic thyroid cancer, which kills nearly 100 percent of its victims within six months of diagnosis.

The word *tumor* refers to *any* lump or growth, and makes no statement as to whether the growth is benign or malignant. Some "benign" tumors are capable of causing death by virtue of growth in a critical place, for example in the brain; but, in general, benign tumors are nonlethal, and malignant tumors are those which are potentially lethal. We use three primary criteria to determine whether tissue is malignant: (1) degree of differentiation, (2) invasion, and (3) ability to metastasize. Using these three criteria, we can classify any growth, including those occurring in the breast.

ALL THOSE CANCERS LOOK ALIKE

When a pathologist looks at a slice of tissue under the micro-scope, he can tell you, without knowing where it came from, whether the tissue he is looking at is from the breast, bone, heart, lungs, lymph nodes, liver, and so on. Each of the body's tissues has specific cell characteristics by which it can be identified. The various types of cells are *differentiated* from any other cell types. When cells multiply at an abnor-mal rate, they can lose some of their specific characteristics and begin to lack differentiation. Such cells are often dis-ordered in arrangement, and it becomes difficult to tell their tissue of origin. This loss of differentiation, or *anaplasia*, is characteristic of malignant cells. Malignant breast tissue looks different from normal breast tissue, and in fact some cells can become so completely undifferentiated, or anaplastic, that the pathologist may not be able to identify them unless he is told exactly where in the body the tissue was located. He could identify the tissue as malignant by the anaplasia, but in very anaplastic tumors he might not be able to tell you the tissue of origin (for example, breast vs. intestine).

In malignant tumors, growth is occurring so rapidly that one can see many cells caught in the process of division (mitosis)—something seen less often in tissues growing at the slower, normal rate. There is a correlation between the degree of anaplasia and the aggressiveness of the malignancy—well-differentiated malignant tumors tend to be less aggressive and less lethal, while anaplastic, or poorly differentiated, tumors tend to grow and spread more rapidly.

KNOWING ONE'S PLACE

The second determinant of malignancy is *invasion*. Benign tis-sues tend to remain within well-defined borders, sometimes even inside a capsule. They may press against adjacent normal tissue, but they do not penetrate at the microscopic cellular level. Malignant tumors, however, can be seen to penetrate and invade neighboring structures, both grossly (with the naked eye) and microscopically. Invasion, in fact, is all that is needed to diagnose what may otherwise look like a benign growth as malignant. In other words, under our first criterion, differentiation, the tumor might look quite benign, but it may still have to be classified as malignant because it has "invaded" surrounding structures; though the cells may maintain an orderly appearance, they have breeched their assigned geographical boundary.

It is this invasion, combined with metastasis (as defined below) and further invasion that ultimately leads to the death of the patient.

THERE GOES THE NEIGHBORHOOD

Benign tumor cells are incapable of leaving their original positions to take up residence at new locations. They can grow only where they originate, while malignant tumors have the capability of *metastasis*, growth at a distant site. Cells may break off, travel via the bloodstream or lymphatic circulation, and begin to grow as a new focus of malignancy elsewhere. It is this capability to metastasize that gives most malignancies their lethality. Breast cancer, for example, has little opportunity to kill while it is localized in the area of the breast, because the breast has no life-support function. It is the growth of metastatic breast cancer in vital organs (for example, the liver, lung, or brain) that will eventually kill the patient. So understanding metastasis is a very important part of understanding cancer itself. It is in its potential for invasion and metastasis that cancer's major lethality exists.

An interesting example of one of the secrets of malignancy lies in the regeneration capability of the human liver. One can remove 80 percent of a human liver (for example, after a gunshot wound or an auto injury) and the liver that remains will begin to regenerate. It will grow to its original size, weight, and approximate shape. While it is regenerating, the growth rate will vastly exceed that of almost any malignant tumor, yet somehow the liver knows when and where to stop. It does not invade. It does not metastasize. It is in every way behaving as a benign growth. Wherever this incredible and mysterious biological control resides, it is precisely this control that makes a growth benign. Unfortunately, we still do not know why loss of control develops in some tissue growth and not in others. Therein lies the fundamental secret of cancer.

It is important to keep in mind the difference between what we refer to as the *primary tumor* and the metastasis. This difference has caused confusion among the lay public. People often say someone died of "liver cancer," when in fact the patient may have had a cancer of the rectum as his "primary." What this means is that cells composed of tissue arising in the rectum lost their original characteristics (became anaplastic, or poorly differentiated), grew through the rectal wall (invasion), and finally spread via the bloodstream to the liver (metastasis). There the abnormal growth became lethal by compromising the liver's function. What is important to remember is that this is a rectal cancer at its inception, and when it moves to the liver it is *still* a rectal cancer growing in the liver. Again, if it is not too undifferentiated, or anaplastic, the pathologist could look at a tissue specimen taken from this metastasis in the liver and tell the clinician that he is dealing with the colon or rectal carcinoma metastatic to the liver. It is not a "primary liver cancer."

BREAST CANCER

With the exception of the lens of the eye and the teeth, virtually any cell in the body may undergo change and assume an aberrant form of growth. In such a case, cell differentiation is lost, growth restraint disappears, and invasion and metastasis follow. The patient has cancer. How then is breast cancer different? What causes it? Who can expect to get it?

Before delving into specific aspects of breast malignancy, it is necessary to understand a few basics of normal breast anatomy. The female breast is a familiar structure, present in a multiplicity of sizes and shapes. From a surgical point of view, however, it is the surrounding anatomy which is important in terms of localization of disease spread. The breast rests against the chest wall, and immediately underlying the breast is the large, fan-shaped pectoralis major muscle. This is covered with a sheath of connective tissue (fascia) that separates the breast from the underlying muscle. This fascia forms an important barrier to the initial spread of the cancer and will be discussed further in connection with surgical treatment. The muscle traverses the chest wall to insert in the upper portion of the arm. This is significant because, in the classic radical mastectomy, this muscle was removed in order to get wide margins around the cancer. The pectoralis major muscle is generally no longer removed, since removal has been found to add little to the cure rate, and since a more normal-looking postoperative appearance and better arm function can be obtained with the modern operation, the "modified" radical mastectomy, or "total" mastectomy.

The female breast is a gland with a cellular structure capable of producing secretions (for example, milk during lactation) which can be directed through channels or ducts which join like tributaries of a river and exit through small openings in the nipple. Over 80 percent of all breast cancers arise from the cells which line these ducts (*ductal* carcinomas). The male breast, while not capable of the structural and functional changes which occur in the female breast, does have ducts and is also capable of forming ductal carcinomas. In fact, of all breast carcinomas, approximately 1 percent occur in males. However, breast carcinoma has rarely been reported in children prior to puberty. While ductal carcinomas are the most common type of breast cancer, there are also less common forms which arise from other structures within the breast. For example, the breast is divided into small lobules of secretory cells structured like bunch grapes which drain into ducts, and these cells can form *lobular* carcinomas. These have a biological behavior slightly different from that of the typical ductal carcinoma, in that there is a higher incidence of simultaneous occurrence in the opposite breast.

WHY ME?

In the study of any form of cancer, one first looks for the cause (etiology). For example, the most widely recognized causal relationship is that of cigarette smoking and lung cancer, despite the shrill protestations of the tobacco industry to the contrary. We do not have such a single specific cause or agent in the case of carcinoma of the breast. There are factors in the family history which tend to put certain patients in a higher or lower risk group, but as yet, no single specific agent has been found.

Carcinoma of the breast is the most common malignant tumor in women in the Western world. In America the disease will strike about 7 percent of white females and approximately 6 percent of black females, with an overall mortality of approximately 23 percent. The more optimistic way of expressing these statistics is that 93 to 94 percent of American women will probably *not* develop breast cancer, and of the remaining 6 to 7 percent who do, 77 percent can expect to be cured. The incidence of breast carcinoma increases with age, with 75 percent of tumors occurring in patients over 50 years old and 50 percent occurring in those over 65.

This general incidence of breast cancer in American women (6 to 7 percent) increases among relatives of patients with *unilateral postmenopausal* breast cancer to about 10 percent, and among relatives of patients with *unilateral premenopausal* breast cancer to about 20 percent. Direct family members of patients with *bilateral postmenopausal* breast cancer have an incidence of almost 28 percent. Though a strong family history definitely increases the chances of developing breast cancer, the exact genetic determinant is unknown. Thus a positive family history, while not an absolute indication that one will develop breast cancer, still places the patient in the group of women who must be closely watched and examined.

Other factors in the total risk of developing breast cancer are less clear. Women in countries where the fat content of the diet is low, such as Japan or Korea, have a strikingly lower incidence of breast cancer than in countries where fat intake is higher. This appears to be an environmental rather than a genetic factor. When these same Asian peoples migrate to Western countries and increase their fat intake, or when they increase their fat intake in their own countries, the incidence of breast carcinoma increases rapidly enough to be evident even within the migrating generation. This may be related to a high dietary content of steroids (structurally related to female sex hormones), which are used to fatten cattle and are introduced into the Western diet through fatty meats. On the genetic side, the disease is definitely more prevalent in white Jewish women.

The exact relation of female sex hormones to breast cancer is also not entirely clear. It appears that lifetime exposure to estrogen increases the risk of developing cancer and that women who, for various reasons, have had their ovaries removed before the age of 35 have a markedly lower risk. There is some evidence that the action of the reproductive hormones in women who have their first pregnancies before the age of 20 may reduce the incidence of carcinoma of the breast, while those women who have their first children after the age of 40 have five times the risk of the younger mothers. While it was originally thought that lactation, nursing, and a higher number of pregnancies decreased the chance of developing breast cancer, more recent studies have shown that this may merely be a statistical artifact.

Although these factors have some bearing on general risk and incidence in the development of breast cancer, we have all seen patients who have had no prior family history, who come from countries in which a low-fat diet is prevalent, who have had early pregnancies, and who have developed breast cancer. At the same time, there are patients with strong family histories and all of the high risk factors who have not developed breast cancer. These risk factors are only clues which should raise the physician's index of suspicion as to which women require more careful scrutiny and more frequent examination. This closer follow-up can bring the disease to our attention at an earlier and possibly more curable stage.

Early detection is at this time still our main weapon of attack against this disease. Weekly or even daily self-examination (see Appendix B) and annual or semiannual examination by a physician are still the mainstays of early diagnosis. Specific modes of diagnosis will be discussed later in detail.

The most common presenting symptom for breast cancers is the "lump." Most lumps are found by the patient herself (like Lucy) or by the examining physician. The most common difficulty encountered during self-examination is the differentiation of an important, possibly cancerous lump from those other, benign lumps which normally appear in the breast. More than 90 percent of women in the premenopausal age group have numerous small cysts (little sacs of fluid), which are usually of no consequence. Very recently it has been found that these cysts seem to be prevalent in women who have a high intake of foods containing chemicals called methylxanthines. Coffee, tea, dark colas, and chocolate are all high in methylxanthine content, and many women who suffer from "cystic breasts" seem to undergo marked reduction in the size and number of these cysts simply by eliminating the methylxanthine-containing foods from their diets. There has never been a proven relationship between cystic disease of the breast and cancer of the breast, but the presence of these cysts often makes life difficult for both the patient and the doctor, because large, firm cysts may have to be biopsied to prove that they are not, in fact, actually cancers. Furthermore, these cysts tend to become painfully engorged with fluid (mastodynia) just prior to the menstrual cycle and are the cause of much suffering for which there is really no adequate treatment. How then does one determine whether the lump is significant? This is a difficult problem. The experience and skill of the examining physician are, of course, the major diagnostic tools. Therefore, any lump that is *different* from the others, that stands out and makes itself known by its different feel, should be a signal to the patient for further examination.

During pregnancy the breasts enlarge, becoming engorged with fluid and secretions, and in most cases feel much more "lumpy" than the nonpregnant breast. It is, therefore, much more difficult to detect a carcinoma in the pregnant patient, and delay in diagnosis may be prolonged for many months, until the pregnancy is over. It is often in the immediate post-partum period, when the breasts begin to return to normal size, that the carcinoma is discovered. Furthermore, the high levels of estrogens present in pregnancy may stimulate growth of the cancer and may necessitate a decision as to whether or not to terminate the pregnancy.

A rarer form of presentation is what is known as *Paget's disease* of the nipple. This involves ductal carcinomas which may be too small to be felt but from which cells have migrated up into the nipple. These microscopic nests of tumor cells in the skin cause itching, redness, and soreness of the nipple. The diagnosis is made in this case by taking a biopsy of the nipple skin to look for cancerous cells. Paget's disease always signals the presence of a primary ductal carcinoma somewhere in the substance of the involved breast and is treated in the same way as any other ductal carcinoma, with a very high cure rate. However, not all rashes or itching of the nipple are the result of Paget's disease.

Another classification known as *inflammatory* carcinoma occurs when the lymphatics and vessels become plugged with tumor and the breast becomes reddened, thickened, tender to the touch, and has all the appearances of infection. This type of carcinoma is particularly lethal because of the rich blood supply and the rapidity of spread. Treatment for this type of carcinoma will be discussed in a later chapter.

The next large category of breast cancer is *lobular* carcinoma. This is less common but still has potential for invasion, spread, and lethality. Lobular carcinomas can be bilateral and one must carefully examine the opposite breast for a "mirror image" carcinoma. Often symmetrical biopsies are performed when a primary carcinoma of the lobular type is found in one breast, even though no lump is felt in the other.

The remaining forms of breast cancer are much less common. These include *tubular* carcinoma, malignant *cystosarcoma phylloides*, *medullary* carcinoma, *adenoid cystic* carcinoma, and several other even rarer types. These are important only to the pathologist and their treatment and diagnosis are still governed by many of the same rules that apply to ductal or lobular carcinomas.

THE PRINCESS AND THE PEA

Not all lumps of the breast are carcinomas, and in fact the vast majority of lumps brought to the attention of the physician are benign. Common fluid-filled cysts must be examined and differentiated from carcinomas. *Fibroadenoma* is a hard, benign tumor which has no potential for malignant change and is removed for diagnosis and sometimes for cosmetic reasons. *Sclerosing adenosis* is a benign disease, but microscopically it can be difficult to differentiate from a carcinoma. A skilled pathologist should be able to make this diagnosis and prevent an unnecessary mastectomy. *Intraductal papilloma* is a polyp of ductal tissue within the duct system of the breast and there is some confusion regarding its propensity to transform into a cancer. The usual symptom is bloody nipple discharge with no palpable lump. All bleeding nipple discharge must be investigated by biopsy to rule out the presence of carcinoma within the polyp, despite the fact that the vast majority of these will turn out to be benign.

The most plaguing question of all has not yet been resolved: What is a precancerous lesion, or what lesions do indeed turn into cancer if left over a long period of time? A homily among breast cancer surgeons is that the most common precancerous lesion of the breast is a carcinoma in the opposite breast. Patients who develop carcinoma in one breast have a much higher risk of developing a new carcinoma in the opposite breast in later years.

Thus the structure of the breast is the birthplace of both benign and malignant growth. In spite of the lack of a single, clear-cut etiologic agent leading to the development of breast cancer, there are several factors which place certain women in a category of higher risk than the general population. Early detection is still our most powerful tool, and this brings us to the specific diagnostic procedures which follow the discovery of the suspicious "lump."

3

Is It
Cancer?

Lucy

New Year's Eve. I was taking a shower, thinking idly of the party we were going to that night. Soaping myself, I felt the lump in my breast. My heart seemed to stop as I ran my fingers over my left breast again, hoping it was my imagination. But there was something there. Just a small bump — I felt hot and my legs were weak — there was definitely a lump.

I dried myself slowly. My fingers kept returning to my breast. I looked in the mirror. Maybe I was mistaken. I felt again. There. It was there — foreign, intrusive, ugly. A lump.

I didn't tell Jack. It was New Year's Eve and I didn't want to spoil the holiday. That's what I told myself. But, truthfully, I couldn't make myself say the hateful words out loud. If I didn't talk about it, maybe it would go away.

I had a new dress for the party. It was made of soft, clinging velvet, cut very low in the front; so low that I had a new bra which made my breasts swell outward through the décolletage. At first self-conscious, and finally flushed with vanity, I preened for Jack. As he admired me, I thought of the lump. How ironic that tonight I offered my breasts for approbation.

And the entire evening, while we laughed and drank and celebrated, I thought about the lump. I found myself on the couch next to Harold, whom I knew very casually. Harold, sodden with holiday joy, was exclaiming the merits of my exposed bosom, especially the left one — the left one had the lump. With a scornful laugh, I told him it was his. He could have the lump, too. Later, sitting quietly with my cousin Margaret, we talked, as we often did, of the charmed lives we had led. Both of us had good marriages. Both of us had healthy, bright children. Both of us had a sense of personal worth. Nothing untoward had happened to us. Whenever we had this conversation we began by listing our advantages and then continued to wonder how long we would be allowed to know nothing but blessings. It was a maudlin dialogue but usually it was reinforcing. This night, I mouthed the words while my thoughts ricocheted and echoed in my mind. The lump. The lump. The lump.

New Year's Day passed. It was silly to tell Jack on New Year's Day. What could be done about it on New Year's Day? But my mood was obvious. And he questioned my quietness and my withdrawal.

Finally, the next evening, I told him. It had been difficult living two days with the secret and I needed to share my fear. He wanted to see the lump, and, after feeling it, thought it too small to be so concerned. Neither of us knew what too small was. He was shaken by my terror, but he was practical; always practical. At that point, a pattern was established — whenever I was tearful and afraid, Jack became hopeful and tenacious. When he was full of despair, I calmed and became the comforter.

The following morning I saw our internist. "It probably isn't anything," he said after he examined me, "but I'd like you to see a surgeon." A surgeon! I didn't know any surgeons. Jack and I had been married for fifteen years and had had three children. We had made wills with appointed guardians in case of a common disaster. But, believing nothing could ever really happen to us, we had never bothered to consider a surgeon.

I asked our doctor to recommend someone and he gave me a list of three names. In a hurried conversation, we discussed them with Jack. We knew all three socially and finally chose one because he had been trained at the finest schools and hospitals, because his reputation was excellent, and because he was young. An appointment was made for me to see him immediately.

Again I lay on an examining table, counting the holes in each square of acoustical ceiling tile. The surgeon palpated my breast. He asked me to sit up; raise my arms; stretch them to the front; to the sides; lean over. He was calm. He was comforting. He confirmed that there was indeed a lump in my breast and there was also a dimpling that might imply a malignancy. He carefully explained that if it were malignant he might be able to excise a wedge from my breast, but added, reassuringly, that it would fill in quickly and not be noticeable for long. I don't remember hearing the word mastectomy; either that it was indicated or that it was even a possibility. There is no doubt, because of the condition of the breast, that the surgeon did discuss the option. There is also no doubt that I denied that reality. I had begun protecting myself.

Mutely, I listened to the surgeon reserve a room in the hospital for that afternoon. I drove home, told Jack what was planned, and arranged for the children to stay with my mother. Fourteen-year-old Ken, Rob, eleven, and Cathy, ten, were interested but not overly concerned when I explained that I had a lump in my breast and had to go to the hospital for surgery. I assured them they shouldn't worry and that I would probably be home in a few days. They were far more anxious about whether they still had to go to Sunday school tomorrow.

My calmness was a lie. I wanted to scream and kick and deny what was happening to me. But instead I made rules. I had to act "maturely." I had to be "brave and uncomplaining." I had to set the tone for the family. I had to be a "good sport." And I denied my feelings. I denied that I felt manipulated and rushed, just as I had denied the thought of a mastectomy. I was encapsulated in a membrane of fear and loneliness.

I knew nothing about breast cancer. In spite of the fact that my grandmother, my mother, and my aunt had had mastectomies, I was ignorant of the disease. Because these women had not died of cancer, and because I was terrified by the thought of it happening to me, it was easy to keep pushing the possibility back. I had never examined my breasts regularly. Illness frightened me. Doctors awed me. Hospitals overwhelmed me.

That afternoon, getting ready to go to the hospital, was a time of absolute terror. As I packed my suitcase, I found the letters and jottings which I had been writing since college. I stopped and thumbed through them. They were brief but each one brought back a time, an emotion, an attitude. I could read four lines and remember what I had been feeling, if the day was sunny, who said what, and my reaction to it. The writing was raw and unadorned. So much of it involved anger, disappointment, frustration. What if something happened to me? What if Jack came home from my funeral and found them? Would he think I had been unhappy always? Why hadn't I written more about the happy times? Last summer was so perfect. We had learned to play tennis and it was a time of sharing. Just the two of us. We ate when we wanted and played when we wanted and time wasn't important except that there be enough of it for us to do what we wanted. Why hadn't I written more about times like last summer? Not wanting those stark words to be my legacy, I threw my precious scribblings in the garbage can, afraid that my honesty would be destructive. I denied myself again. I hadn't learned yet that self-denial is the most destructive force of all.

I went into the hospital on a Saturday. I was scheduled for surgery on Monday morning. When I had protested spending the weekend in bed in the hospital, the surgeon had soothed me by explaining that if I didn't take the room when it was available I might not be able to get one on Monday. And because we were unprepared, I docilely let myself be led into the hospital for two wasted days. Wasted time. Wasted money. Wasted space. We watched television. Friends visited. We talked of trivial things: which team would win the Super Bowl; a party the following weekend. We walked the halls, trying not to look into other people's lives, but looking anyway. We talked about the children. We talked of how we loved each other. We never spoke of illness or dying. But I thought about it constantly. If Jack were having the same thoughts, he never verbalized them either. We protested we were confident of a benign diagnosis.

I was subjected to various tests: blood, urine, x-ray. All of them could have been done in a two-hour period. Instead, because I was there, it took two days. The anesthesiologist came to my room to explain what type of anesthetic would be used. The surgeon came to tell me the time of the operation and to assure me that there was no need to worry. Again, I don't remember hearing either man mention the word mastectomy. But then, I didn't mention it either.

There wasn't much more to say. Jack left knowing that I would probably be sedated when he saw me the next morning on my way to the operating room. I stood at the window watching him walk across the parking lot. The light standards cast a very long shadow and I waved forlornly, wishing my shadow were side by side with his. And because it was my way, I started writing down my thoughts again.

Journal Excerpt—January, 1970

It's five o'clock in the morning and I can't sleep. I'm scared. And I'm lonely—me, who can handle everything by myself, who doesn't need people . . . maybe because I've always had the choice. It's too early to call anyone and the nurses are too busy for idle conversation. Here I sit . . . can't read . . . just hoping Jack will call when he wakes up. Nighttime is the most frightening and the loneliest. So many questions . . . and I don't want to think about the answers. The hospital strips me of all positive motivation. I lie back and let it happen. But the sky is getting lighter. Jack will be here soon.

When Jack arrived, the rest of the family was gathered in the hall outside my room. I had told them that I wanted no one with me but Jack. The shot was already taking effect and I feared being out of control in front of anyone—anyone but Jack. We talked. He promised me I would never have to have a private nurse. We had seen so many as we walked around the hospital. I hated the thought of a stranger with me day and night. I wanted privacy. We held hands. I wanted to protect him. He wanted to protect me. We could only say, again and again, "I love you." And then I was being moved through the hall. I felt him kiss me and fade away.

Detached, I watched the activity outside the operating room. A surgeon in his green suit waved to me and turned to blow his nose in his hand. I flinched—and flinched again at the bright chatter from the orderlies and nurses about their night-before activities. No one seemed aware or concerned that I was facing the most important event of my life.

The anesthesiologist swabbed my arm and cheerfully explained he would be injecting sodium pentathol, which would make me sleep. I counted backwards for him. . . .

It hurt. I wanted to move but my arm was taped to my body. I tried to answer when I heard someone call my name, but I could only ask, "What happened? Do I have cancer? Is my breast still there?" My mouth was thick. The nurse clucked and fussed. "You'll be fine. Your doctor will talk to you and answer all your questions. Just rest and your *own* nurse will be here to take you back to your room." Your *own* nurse. *My* nurse? A private nurse. Jack had said no—he wouldn't. And he wouldn't. Unless. . . .

And so I knew.

Tony

Lucy found a lump in her breast. To her doctor, it felt highly suspicious. It was promptly biopsied and cancer was found. On physical examination it may be very difficult for the patient, and sometimes for the examining physician, to determine which lumps call for biopsy and which lumps do not. Because the vast majority of women have numerous small lumps within the breast, it is necessary to determine which of these need biopsy. If we were to biopsy every woman who appeared in the office with a "lump," we would do four or five biopsies a day, to the exclusion of all other surgery. More important, many women would undergo unnecessary surgery. On the other hand, we like to make the diagnosis in cases of cancer as early as possible. The most important single determinant is the presence of a lump or a mass which has not been present previously and which stands out when compared to the rest of the lumps of the breast. In general, most breasts feel uniformly nodular, with little variation in the size or hardness of the lumps. The presence of one which is different from the rest indicates the need for further examination.

COMMENDABLE ASPIRATIONS

The majority of the lumps found in the breast are benign, probably in a ratio of ten or more to one, depending on the age of the population of patients being examined. Most of these will be simple cysts, and in many cases the diagnosis can be made by inserting a needle into the mass and aspirating (withdrawing) the fluid. However, there are certain rules which must be followed to avoid missing a carcinoma when doing a needle aspiration. First, the withdrawal of the fluid should be followed by *complete* disappearance of the mass.

If there is any residual mass present, this, in itself, is an indication for tissue biopsy. In many cases, future reaspiration of fluid may be necessary, and surgeons generally feel that persistent reaccumulations and the need for reaspirations also warrant biopsy. The exact number of needle aspirations permissible in any one patient has not been established.

Some investigators feel that the presence of blood in the aspirated fluid indicates the need for biopsy, and although this is probably a safe rule to follow, in most cases the blood will be secondary to the insertion of the needle itself. There is still some debate as to whether all aspirated fluid should be sent for microscopic examination to determine if malignant cells are present. The overwhelming majority of cysts are benign, and the chance of finding malignant cells within these cysts is exceptionally small, even in the presence of carcinomas. The cost involved in sending all cyst fluid for microscopic examination may indeed be prohibitive, considering the very few carcinomas that will be found with this technique.

Thus a great many lumps can be securely diagnosed as benign cysts through fine needle aspirations alone, and as long as we are willing to biopsy *all* those lumps which do not completely disappear, as well as those from which no fluid is obtained (suggesting a solid mass rather than a fluid-filled cyst), we are on acceptably safe ground and should not be afraid of missing a carcinoma.

On occasion, failure to aspirate fluid will lead to open biopsy and only a cyst will be found. This is generally due to the fact that aspiration is a "blind" technique, carried out by feel, and the needle will sometimes miss the cyst. In such a case, only open biopsy will give a sure diagnosis.

The vast majority of carcinomas are diagnosable the first time they are felt, and an experienced surgeon or physician should have an accuracy of diagnosis somewhere in the 90 to 95 percent range merely by palpating the lump.

Some of the characteristics of a typical carcinoma include irregular shape, extreme firmness or hardness, and the sensation that it is fixed to the surrounding tissues (invasion). The more advanced carcinomas may be fixed to the underlying muscle or skin, and carcinoma which extends microscopically up through the lymphatics into the skin may cause the skin to be dimpled in numerous small areas, resembling the skin of a coarse orange (known in French and in medical parlance as "peau d'orange"). Finally, traction on the skin may cause actual dimpling of the skin or inversion of the nipple. This is best demonstrated by having the patient raise her arms above her head, accentuating the dimpling by the downward countertraction of the breast. Although some women have one-sided nipple inversion throughout their lives, any nipple which becomes newly inverted in adult life must be considered to harbor a carcinoma until proven otherwise. Physical examination of the armpit (axilla) also indicates a need for further investigation if the lymph nodes are enlarged and firm — normal lymph nodes are small and soft enough to be undetectable by routine palpation. Itching or scaliness with redness around the nipple is seen in Paget's disease and may indicate an underlying carcinoma whether any lump is felt or not.

After the complete physical examination and evaluation of the lump by the patient and the physician, an immediate decision can usually be made as to whether biopsy should be undertaken. When the patient is young and has no family history of breast cancer, and if the mass itself is not suggestive of a breast cancer, it is sometimes preferable to follow the patient at intervals of several weeks to see if there is any change. Although no patient with a breast cancer should be unduly delayed in diagnosis and treatment, delays of up to several weeks do no harm to the patient. Although for most women the presence of a lump is a psychological emergency, the diagnosis and treatment do not constitute a medical emergency. It is estimated that anywhere from three to five years may elapse between the time the first cancer cell arises in the breast and the time the tumor is large enough to be felt (when it is about the size of a pea). Therefore, delays of weeks or even months may be of no clinical significance. Following the patient along for a short period of time may avoid unnecessary breast biopsy. It is also helpful at times to examine the premenopausal patient during a different time in the menstrual cycle, because breast cysts tend to become enlarged just prior to the onset of the menstrual period and may be much smaller in mid-cycle. This size variation does not occur with carcinomas. Therefore, one may delay a biopsy from two to six weeks in order to reexamine the patient at a completely different hormonal time. Obviously, in the case of the suspicious lump an expeditious scheduling for biopsy is required.

THE MISUNDERSTOOD MAMMOGRAM

Before describing the techniques of and the alternatives to biopsy, we should discuss one of the most commonly used and misused diagnostic tools in all of medicine: the mammogram. X-rays of the breast for carcinoma have been available for many years. There are few subjects in medicine that have evoked so much debate and misunderstanding among both the lay public and the physicians who order and interpret the tests. In general, mammograms are safe, noninvasive x-rays of the breast which may show up small carcinomas at an early, and therefore more curable, stage. At the present time, the most commonly used forms are the Xeromammogram and the conventional x-ray mammogram. Both of these tests involve low-dose radiation and should not present any health hazard in the form of induction of cancer. The public's generally unfounded fear that mammograms may lead to carcinomas has been detrimental to the diagnostic and clinical value of these studies.

Today's low-dose mammography techniques can involve as little as 0.03 rad, which dose is negligible when balanced against its usefulness in detecting early cancers (this is discussed at greater depth in Chapter 4). The judicious use of mammograms in detecting small carcinomas far outweighs the risk of developing carcinoma from mammogram radiation.

However, the most misunderstood aspect is the fact that the mammogram is no more accurate than palpation of the breast when the lump has already been felt. Once a lump is present and palpated, the mammogram has a 15 percent margin of error in producing both false negatives and false positives, whereas with physical examination alone the accuracy may be in the 90 percent range. Therefore, the mammogram is not a great additional help in such instances. The mammogram's most effective use is primarily for the localization of very small carcinomas that cannot otherwise be palpated. The reason for ordering a mammogram prior to the biopsy is not to increase diagnostic accuracy, since the suspicious lump is going to be biopsied regardless of what the mammogram shows, but to see if there are any *other* lumps that have not been *felt* but which may be even more suspicious on x-ray and should be biopsied at the same time as the palpable lumps.

When small nonpalpable areas suspicious for carcinoma are present on the mammogram, several techniques can be used to localize them at the time of biopsy. Under local anesthesia, a needle can sometimes be inserted into the suspicious area under x-ray control, and when the needle is seen to be at or in the mass, a small amount of blue dye can be injected. This allows the surgeon to go directly to the area of the blue dye and to avoid removing more breast tissue than is necessary. When a suspicious area is seen on the mammogram (sometimes marked by tiny flecks of calcium), the tissue specimen can be sent to radiology first and x-rayed to make sure the proper tissue has been removed. The appearance of small calcium particles on the x-ray of the specimen is proof that the suspicious area has indeed been located.

Mammography's usefulness increases in the older patient as more of the breast tissue is replaced by fat, allowing the remaining breast tissue to stand out in contrast. Conversely, in the younger patient there is less fat and more dense breast tissue, making mammograms harder to interpret. The x-ray becomes virtually useless in teenagers and should not be used because of its lack of diagnostic value as well as the extreme rarity of breast cancer below the age of twenty.

THERMOGRAPHY

There are still a few strong proponents of thermography, a technique which measures the heat emission from areas of the breast. Thermography detects cancer through the increased blood supply of a malignant tumor, but this has not been proven to be any more helpful or more accurate than the combined use of mammography and physical examination. In fact, at this time thermography has been virtually abandoned in clinical practice, except at a few isolated centers. The only virtues are its lack of any radiation output and its noninvasive nature.

BIOPSY TECHNIQUES

We should recognize that biopsy with examination of the tissue under the microscope is the *only* definitive procedure upon which further treatment can be based. However, the most difficult of decisions is which lumps need to be biopsied, and which may be safely followed by serial examination and left in place.

It would be wonderful to believe that your physician can do no wrong—after all it is your health and sometimes life in his hands—but the reality is that infallibility is beyond human capability.

The Lump Stops Here

This burden is most heavy for the surgeon dealing with the breast lump. For the surgeon who evaluates this patient, the entire responsibility is his. Patients may be screened by their gynecologist or family physician, but those doctors can always opt to pass the burden on to the general surgeon by referring the case to him. And "the lump stops there."

It would be easy (though a bad idea) to merely biopsy every lump presented for evaluation. Then the surgeon would never have to fear missing a possible carcinoma. But, in fact, the vast majority of lumps turn out to be benign, and countless women would be subjected to unnecessary surgery, expense, and possible danger. So, we must select those whose lumps are more suspicious from those whose lumps are not, and that is the most difficult of decisions.

That's Why They Put Erasers on Pencils

My 12-year-old daughter, Katie, was upset when she found out that I had misinformed her on the origins of pizza. She had had an argument at school with her classmates and teacher, and used "my daddy" as her reference. When sent to the library to settle the argument, she returned corrected, and disappointed that her daddy could be wrong. When she told me the story I was, at first, sad that I had let her down. But after thinking about it for a bit I told her that perhaps this was a good time to find out that even I could make mistakes. I was confident she'd love me anyway. Once she understood that I, too, was only human, she'd be less likely to have to face that disappointment later. The longer that the realization of my fallibility was delayed, the more difficult it would be for her to accept.

The decision *not* to biopsy is the difficult one, and it must be made by a fallible human being. Without being overly dramatic, that is a heavy responsibility, and while we all like to feel we've evaluated every source of information, there is still no surgeon who feels entirely easy about sending the patient away without biopsy proof of a benign diagnosis.

Needle Aspiration

The least intrusive type of biopsy is needle aspiration. Fine needle aspiration biopsy is a safe procedure and can be performed under local anesthesia in the doctor's office. The area of the breast under question is swabbed with antiseptic, a very thin needle is inserted into the lump, and cells from the lump are drawn into the syringe by suction. This tissue is sprayed onto a slide (in much the same manner as a "Pap" smear) and examined under a microscope for malignant cells.

Similar to this is the larger needle biopsy in which a cutting needle is inserted into the mass and a slice of breast tissue is taken and sent for microscopic examination. These biopsies can be performed in the office and present no hazard to the patient and relatively little pain. The old fear that tumor cells might be injected along the tract of the needle has not been borne out in practice, and widespread dissemination of malignancy has not been found to be a danger with this procedure. The major drawback to needle aspiration is that a negative result does not always mean there is no cancer present. The needle may simply have missed the area of cancer. Thus one can see that needle biopsy is mainly advantageous with those tumors that are highly suspicious, in that it gives the physician a chance to do a biopsy and prepare the patient for surgery prior to actually going into the operating room. This will also eliminate the extra operating time and expense involved in doing an inpatient biopsy under anesthesia.

Incisional Biopsy

The next type of biopsy is known as *incisional* biopsy, whereby a piece of the tumor is taken. This type of biopsy is usually reserved for very large tumors which cannot be surgically removed and which will probably be treated by radiation and chemotherapy. Incisional biopsy is used in these cases to prove the diagnosis so that treatment can be started.

Excisional Biopsy

By far the most commonly used biopsy is the *excisional* biopsy. In this case the entire lump is removed and examined, either by rapid section, in which the tissue is frozen so that a thin slice can be cut for microscopic examination, or by permanent paraffin technique, in which the tissue is imbedded in wax before being sliced for examination. The debate here is whether these biopsies should be done as inpatient or outpatient procedures, or whether a local or general anesthetic should be used. Once again, this depends upon the health of the patient and the index of suspicion for carcinoma.

The least costly method to the patient, both financially and psychologically, is to biopsy the lump with local anesthesia on an outpatient basis and await the examination of the permanent paraffin sections of the biopsy before proceeding further with treatment.

When suspicion is high, most physicians would prefer to have the patient asleep and prepared for surgical treatment at the time of biopsy. The lump is then removed and sent for microscopic examination (frozen section). If a definitive diagnosis of cancer is made, the surgeon will proceed at that time with mastectomy or with whatever form of treatment has been agreed upon by the physician and patient prior to the biopsy. Excisional biopsy gives the greatest chance for accurate diagnosis, since the lump is completely removed, and it is the rare case in which definitive diagnosis cannot be made on the frozen section at the time of biopsy. If the microscope slide is difficult to interpret, treatment should always be delayed until other opinions can be obtained. There is no danger in delaying definitive treatment days or even weeks if time is needed to obtain further opinions as to the microscopic diagnosis of cancer.

Breast carcinoma tissue is also examined for estrogen and progesterone receptors at the time of the original biopsy. This is a test which helps in detecting the susceptibility of a specific tumor to treatment with antiestrogen agents or hormonal manipulations.

When the lump is highly suspicious, some physicians will order bone and liver scans to look for metastatic spread of the disease to these organs. These are expensive and time-consuming studies, and most surgeons agree today that, except in the case of obvious carcinomas, these tests can wait until after the initial biopsy is done. In cases where positive findings with these scans would change the course of therapy, then of course the scans should be done first. However, most surgeons believe that the excision of the mass and the breast is still indicated, even in the presence of distant spread, to prevent local recurrence and for other reasons which will be discussed in detail in Chapter 4.

In summary, definitive diagnosis of a lump in the breast is made by excisional biopsy and microscopic examination. Variations exist in the techniques used, depending upon the index of suspicion aroused by physical examination, family history, age, and secondary signs of malignancy. Ancillary examinations (such as mammography) may help in the discovery of other occult carcinomas but should not play a primary role in the diagnosis of the solitary breast lump. The debate over whether mammography should be used as a screening procedure persists, and at this moment its cost-effectiveness in finding early carcinomas is a highly controversial subject. The mainstays of treatment are still frequent self-examination, regular examinations of the breast by the physician, and early biopsy of all suspicious breast masses. Early detection remains the unquestioned mainstay in treatment today.

4

What Do We Do Now?

Lucy

The surgical procedure performed on me was the Halsted radical mastectomy. The surgeon removed my left breast, the axillary lymph nodes, and the pectoral muscle.

I woke up in my room, insisting that, yes, I did indeed want ginger ale. It was dark but I could see Jack sitting hunched in the corner. He didn't say anything. There was a nurse standing on one side of the bed and my sister Betty was standing on the other. It was Betty who gave me the ginger ale. And it was Betty whom I threw up on. She gagged. I giggled. Jack stepped over to my bed. Even in the gloom I could see he looked queasy. I knew how he hated hospitals. And I knew he was scared. Suddenly, I wasn't worried about what had happened to me. I only wanted him to know I was okay. I wanted to touch him. I wanted him to kiss me. I wanted that sick look to disappear from his eyes. I tried to talk but my tongue was thick and the words came out all twisted. It was funny. Jack didn't even smile. It wasn't funny. I had cancer. *Cancer. Oh God, not me. Not cancer. My children are too young. I just learned how to play tennis. I love Jack. I haven't done anything with my life. I'm too young.*

I looked around. My arm was strapped to something. There was a tube in it. Coming out of my chest there were tubes attached to a machine by the bed. My other arm was taped across my body. I felt as if I couldn't move. There was fluid going into me. There was fluid coming out of me. It made gurgling noises. I looked up at Jack and saw his eyes clouded with fear. Fear watching fear. . . .

I woke up again and I was alone. Except for a nurse dozing in a chair. My private nurse. There was no one watching me, no one there who loved me. I could cry. I could feel the pain. I could finally admit what had happened. But the thoughts

tumbled about in my head. I had cancer. I had had a mastectomy. Still, I thought about it abstractly, from a distance,
watching myself. I felt as if I were in a play. I was the star.
How would I act? How should I handle the drama? What was
my role as wife? Mother? Daughter? Sister? Self? Self. . . I
hurt so bad. I had cancer. Nothing mattered but cancer. A
shot. Please, a shot. I didn't want to think any more. Could I
be heroic? A creature to be admired? Would I wallow in pity
for myself? How would Jack act? Would my ugliness repulse
him? Would he feel sorry for me? I felt sorry for me. Oh
hell, I felt so sorry for me. The shot. Now the pain would
go away. . . .

I heard crying. Someone was crying. I wiped my face. It
wasn't me. Someone was crying in the hall. It sounded like
Betty. And then the surgeon strode into my room. Tersely,
he explained that cancer had been found in my lymph nodes
and that I would need radiation treatment.

"Shit," said I.

"You told me you wanted the truth," he said.

Knowing doesn't mean I can't be sad, I screamed silently.
But that brief conversation taught me quickly. *Keep your
feelings to yourself. Deal only with what is real when you
deal with the doctor. He doesn't want to treat emotions.
Only physical reality.* So I denied myself again.

I rationalized that there was no way I could show my real
feelings. Jack came to the hospital to see me every morning
on his way to work and again on his way home. He was
frightened and loving. I was frightened but reassuring. He had
so many pressures — his insurance business, the children, me.
I wanted to relieve some of his anxiety. My brother Dann
came every day, too. He came because he cared, but he
obviously didn't want any ugliness to invade our visit. It was
to be a cheery and pleasant interlude. My sister Betty spent
every day, all day at the hospital. She was good company and
I soon depended on her presence. But she was scared. Scared
for me and scared for herself — what if she got cancer too? I
tried to reassure her. Then there was my mother. I only had
to look at her to see the message in her eyes: Why wasn't it
her? She needed comfort and a reason for living. I worked

hard to ease everyone's heartache and denied my own. I had time to think about myself at night when I was finally, peacefully, terrifyingly alone.

I read and reread the notes the children had sent:

Dear Mom,
I am very sorry on what happened. I know how you feel. Please do not worry we are fine.

XXXXXXX
Love and kisses,
Rob

. . . as soon as I finish this letter I am going to take a bath. Did you have to take a bath? I hope not! I really miss you, that's why I've called you so much.

Love,
Cathy

Dear Mom,
I hope you are feeling better (sorry all I can think of are clichés). You wouldn't believe what bad housekeepers us males are. . . . I send all my love.

Ken

The hospital forbade their visiting me because they were too young. What a stupid rule. But we wrote letters and telephoned. They had been told that I had cancer, because I wanted no secrets. Facts must be faced. Emotions were for hiding. The hospital had its code. I had mine.

Alone, I could not confront the horror of cancer, the mastectomy, my life or death. I allowed the role playing to continue and reacted rather than acted. Other people were making decisions for me, about me. And I let them.

The radiologist came to see me. I questioned him again and again about his qualifications and the course of treatment he had chosen for me. He was unlike the surgeon—less abrupt, less patronizing. He didn't call me "hon" as the surgeon did, and I was grateful for that. The radiologist was frank, open, and honest. He made me feel he had time to spend with me. He didn't frighten me, and I intuitively trusted him. I wanted to believe him when he assured me that the twenty-five radiation treatments he recommended would prevent local recurrence. I was unaware then that if metastasis had already occurred, radiation might be the wrong treatment. The value of nuclear medicine (liver, lung, or bone scan) was not fully realized at that time, nor was such treatment readily available. So, while a bone survey (x-ray) was made, it showed no spread (x-rays are not as effective in detecting metastasis as scanning) and radiation was determined to be the proper treatment. I accepted the determination.

Terrified of radiation, I remembered my father talking of the isolation he felt when he was alone under the ground in a room with the huge cobalt machine. I thought of him often and was glad he didn't have to see me go through the same experience. The hospital provided a bus to take patients to the radiation center. The idea of walking docilely onto a bus to be driven to the darkness of that underground room was abhorrent to me and I insisted that Jack take me, alone, when I was ready to go.

It was like walking into a place for the lost. I don't know if I could have actually stepped through the door if Jack hadn't delivered me directly into the radiologist's hands. I forced my mind to leave my body. I couldn't bear what was happening to me.

Journal Excerpt — January 1970

. . . one doctor, then another and another probe the empty skin place . . . it is so barren my heart makes it move with each beat. They measure and they weigh, and they probe and hit, and pinch bits of tissue between their fingers while I lie there staring at the ceiling, burning with the wish that I were not there. Oh, how I wish I had died in the hospital on the first or second day, when I had yet to realize how much I hated living under this sentence . . . I ooze pity for myself. I am even uglier for it. . . .

I had become a victim. And I was very angry. When the surgeon came to my room to remove the stitches, he brought a retinue of medical students with him (no one had asked if I could be used as a teaching case), and it was depersonalizing.

They marveled over the scar. I thought it hideous—red, scabby, repulsive—but I kept quiet. The surgeon spoke about prostheses. He explained how lifelike they were; they were soft and had fluid motion; you could even buy one with a nipple. I asked him how they tasted. He was embarrassed. I felt better. But I was still angry. When a volunteer from Reach to Recovery asked to see me, I refused.

Reach to Recovery is a marvelous organization peopled by women who have had mastectomies and who are leading useful, busy lives. By their example, a woman newly diagnosed as having breast cancer can learn to cope with her new body; can learn exercises to recover the use of her arm; will be helped to find out where and how to buy the properly fitted prosthesis and where to buy a bathing suit; and can learn how to deal with the emotional trauma of her illness and her mutilation, both with herself and with her family. But I wouldn't allow this information. I didn't want to feel a part of a group of sick people. I would be different. I was different. I knew nothing about my disease, but I was too frightened and angry to admit it. Someone had done something to me and I couldn't trust anyone again. I would have to learn to take care of myself.

When I left the hospital I felt well. The radiation treatments had caused no ill effects so far, and I had begun using my left arm, although it was aching. When I walked into our house, I burst into tears. It was so lovely to be home and I was one step farther from death. Home and children and Jack. Things might be as they were before.

But there was one more hurdle. I had to show Jack my body. I was scared of his reaction, but the need to see his face was greater than my fear. I had to know how he felt right away. He was washing when I walked into the bathroom. I took off my clothes. He looked at me and said, "That's not so bad." And went on washing. I put my nightgown on and waited for him to come to bed. He hadn't grimaced. He hadn't made a joke. He had looked and found it "not so bad." When he got into bed I moved into his arms. I needed him to hold me and to love me. He was afraid he would hurt me but there was no way he could. His love made me know I was still alive. Real. Lucy. The same. We were the same together. I slept.

Journal Excerpt — January, 1970

Jack is wonderful. He, whom I have accused so often of having no empathy, is always standing close behind me — fitting his body, his words, his strengths to mine. How lucky I am.

But my arm began hurting so badly I couldn't sleep, couldn't wash dishes, couldn't even read. We had to find someone to come and take care of the children and the house. No one knew what was causing it. And of course the suspicion was that the cancer had spread. X-rays were made. They showed nothing. An orthopedic man was called in. He found no cause. It was suggested that during my daily radiation treatment the cobalt be aimed at my arm, which would perhaps relieve the pain. It was tried. The pain persisted. But the doctors relaxed about it. They were convinced now that it wasn't fatal, so I was left to deal with it myself — with the help of the codeine, Darvon, Valium, and Seconal that each specialist had prescribed independently. I took it all. Day and night. None of it cured the pain, but I existed in the hazy half light of a drug addict. I could do nothing for myself — except take pills. Every four hours — every two hours — I took the pills. Time had no meaning. Night and day were indiscernible. I lived from pill to pill. I lost the use of my thumb and forefinger. It was agonizing. But I kept taking the pills.

During this time, I was going to the radiation clinic five days a week for treatment. I couldn't drive myself. I was so drugged I couldn't even take a shower by myself. Betty picked me up each morning, drove me to the clinic, waited while I had my treatment, and then drove me home.

I hated the clinic. Everyone was sick and I didn't like thinking of myself that way. I consciously wore my nicest clothes and put on lipstick, trying to set myself apart from the people I saw there — a woman with no nose; a little girl, no more than two, who never smiled and whose eyes were too large and too serious in her shrunken face; men so thin and weak they couldn't walk; women with no hair, wearing scarves to hide their baldness. I spoke to no one. I couldn't be like them. I was afraid that I would soon be like them.

But I still liked the radiologist. He continued to give me his time. He was kind, and honest, and reassuring. Yet he was never condescending. He answered all of my questions and I felt comfortable with him. Because he seemed to care.

I began to think that I was imagining the pain in order to deny that I had cancer. Or maybe I was going crazy. After all, the doctors had still found nothing wrong. Finally, desperately, not knowing where else to turn, Jack took me to a neurologist.

His diagnosis was quick and simple. He found a spur on a bone in my neck and reasoned that when the tube was inserted into my throat during surgery, it damaged a nerve which then affected my arm. His advice was to go back to the hospital into traction. And back I went. He took away all of my pills. Within a week I was better.

So I came home again. But this time, I had no discomfort. I was through with the radiation treatments, which, while not painful, had been debilitating and had slowed the healing of my chest. I had been in traction for ten days. My arm didn't hurt anymore. The process of recuperation had lasted three months.

Now I had time to think about what had happened to me. I knew I had breast cancer. I knew the treatment chosen for me was mastectomy and radiation. I knew my left arm might swell due to the removal of the lymph nodes. And I knew the cancer had metastasized to those lymph nodes. I knew I had to see the surgeon and the radiologist every three months for at least five years. Five years seemed to be the magic time span a cancer patient must live in order to be considered cured. But I knew that wasn't so. I had asked Jack how long it would be before I could buy a life insurance policy, and he had found it would be ten years. Ten years before I would know if I were well. An eternity.

At first, I was happy just to be able to take care of myself and the children. I began playing tennis again. I was strong. I looked healthy. I felt well. But there was always a small voice whispering, "Is it spreading? When will it show up again?" I had no idea what the symptoms would be if there were metastasis. I only knew I was afraid.

Journal Excerpt — July, 1971

Yesterday's newspaper was full of cancer cancer cancer — and quoting about breast cancer, it said, "Once the cancer has spread it is almost always fatal . . . and the spread usually occurs before the cancer is detected in the breast." I just went to pieces and cried and cried — like I knew it but kept hiding from it — and now I can't . . . .

My surgeon suggested I have my remaining breast removed. I was horrified. He explained that when a malignancy is found in one breast the chances are greater it will spread to or appear in the other. I refused. He added that I wasn't so beautiful with only one breast, so what difference could it make? What a son of a bitch. Such an unkind thing to say. I mumbled that I couldn't handle another operation. How could I explain to this brusque man that I wanted to keep my breast if I could. I loved it. It was part of me. I had suffered the loss of one. That was enough. Too much.

What I didn't know then was the extent of my disease. I had asked what kind of cancer I had. "A carcinoma," I was told. "Was it a fast-growing kind?" I had asked. "Probably," was the answer, "but we hope we got it all." I didn't know what else to ask. What had been found was that, of the thirty nodes removed, twenty-three were cancerous — eight nodes in Level I, twelve in Level II, and three in Level III. The surgeon was also concerned because the cancer had metastasized to the lymphatic vessels as well as the nodes. This meant that it could spread very rapidly. I knew none of these details. I never doubted I was being told the truth by the doctors and by Jack. I did sense there was more to be known than what I was aware of, yet I didn't know how to pose the questions. Everything I asked was answered, but I didn't know what to ask.

So I started to read. What was easily available to me were other women's stories of their own experiences with breast cancer. I read them all. When I needed more facts, I borrowed medical texts from my surgeon. As he gave them to me he said, "I wish you wouldn't read these. I'm afraid you'll be frightened." His words frightened me. What was there that I didn't know? What hadn't I been told? I read the books. I became acquainted with muscles and nodes and ducts. I saw pictures of ugly, cancer-ridden breasts. I read of surgical procedures. But I couldn't equate this new knowledge to *me*. I didn't know the medical terms to describe my case. So I seldom identified myself with what I read.

I saw each doctor every three months. I had no pain. There were no new symptoms. My arm swelled, but I learned that if I kept it raised high over my head for two or three hours a day the swelling subsided, and soon I had little problem with it. No doctor had told me to hang it high; another cancer patient had taught me the trick. I took a job. We went to Florida with the children for spring vacation. My life had a routine to it again, a good routine. I had always been a person with mood swings of joy and depression. But now the range was greater. At the top, I was euphoric. I was awed by the sunset, by the love of my friends and family, grateful for every day. When I dropped down, I thought of death, of not seeing my children grown, of a lingering illness. Each time I went for an examination, I fought despair. Every time the x-rays and blood tests were clear, I exulted.

Journal Excerpt — September, 1972

I keep trying to moderate my moods — not soaring quite so high that I don't sink so low — but I don't think that's possible for me. When I'm down I'll try to rise up, but when I'm up I love being up up up, so . . . moderation just isn't me. . . .

Two years had passed. Then three. I was well. I felt smart, omnipotent. I had been right to refuse to have my right breast removed. I didn't want to ever spend time in a hospital again. For progressively longer periods of time I managed to dispel the specter of recurring cancer.

Journal Excerpt — July, 1973

Jack and I are so lucky. If ever the cancer comes back, we have had this time to know what we have and how we feel together. Some people don't ever have that. I always thought it would be best to die quickly — with no warning and no illness. But it's good to have time. It's good to know what loss would be and then not have to lose.

AN ARMED SAVAGE

Lucy wanted facts, but the most definitive statement that one can make about the treatment of breast cancer today is that no definitive statements should be made. Treatment has changed dramatically since my first encounters with the disease as a medical student in the early 1960s and my resident years in the early 1970s. In fact, treatment has changed in a significant fashion in the time interval between the rough draft and the completed version of this book.

John Hunter, one of England's most eminent eighteenth-century surgeons, said: *Surgery is like an armed savage who attempts to get that by force which a civilized man would get by stratagem.*

Unfortunately, 200 years later this is still the case. Surgery should be seen as the worst of all choices of treatment, but one that is still the best we have for many diseases. Breast cancer is one of these diseases.

For almost ninety years, the treatment of breast cancer has been surgical removal of the breast, pectoral muscles, and axillary lymph nodes. This began in the 1890s, when William Halsted of Johns Hopkins introduced the classic radical mastectomy. Among the myriads of innovations that Halsted introduced, radical surgery for cancer of the breast remains one of his greatest contributions, and has for the past ninety years remained the standard against which all other forms of treatment are compared.

Halsted was one of the great geniuses of American surgery. His innovations include the introduction of the use of rubber gloves in surgery, numerous techniques of intestinal suturing, hernia repairs, and, of course, the Halsted radical mastectomy. In fact, his achievements are so numerous that in medical school whenever I was stumped by a question on the history of surgery, I would always answer "Halsted," figuring that the odds alone favored its being the right answer.

It is only in the last fifteen years that his basic technique has been modified at all, and the principles which Halsted elaborated have been only minimally changed. Therefore, discussion of the surgical treatment of breast cancer must necessarily begin with the Halsted radical mastectomy.

The anatomic basis of the radical mastectomy is that of wide surgical excision with removal of the entire breast, the underlying pectoral muscles, and all axillary lymph nodes (see Fig. 1). In practice, this is carried out by making a wide elliptical incision in the skin over the breast cancer, undermining the skin in all directions, and removing all breast tissue. This is performed en bloc, taking the large pectoralis major and minor muscles and then carrying the dissection up into the axilla, removing all levels of the axillary lymph nodes. At the time of Lucy's surgery, most surgeons were still using this technique, and so Lucy began treatment with the classic Halsted radical mastectomy, as had literally millions of breast cancer patients the world over.

The reasons for this radical type of dissection are that it is impossible to detect microscopic spread of the breast cancer within the affected breast and that many breast cancers are multicentric in origin—i.e., there may be more than one microscopic focus of cancer present in the same breast. The rationale for the removal of the large pectoralis major and minor muscles is that this will prevent deep spread of the tumor. Since the axillary lymph nodes are the first line of defense against further tumor spread, it is assumed that they may contain some malignant cells; therefore, these are removed as well. This operation is extremely deforming and cosmetically unacceptable. The removal of the pectoralis major is a prime cause for significant loss in power and function of the arm. The common occurrence of arm swelling after mastectomy stems not from the removal of the lymph nodes draining the breast, but from the enthusiasm of the surgeon who removes the lymph nodes which drain the arm. In the properly executed radical mastectomy, lymph nodes

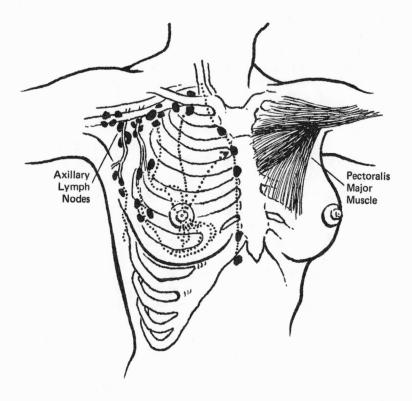

FIGURE 1. The anatomic basis of the radical mastectomy. The entire breast is removed, including the underlying pectoral muscle (shown above on the right) and all axillary lymph nodes (shown above on the left). The lymph nodes are situated under the muscle.

draining the arm will not be removed and swelling should not occur. Some patients will develop arm swelling despite a correct dissection because of the presence of recurrent tumor under the arm, or following the destruction of the remaining lymph nodes which drain the arm by postoperative radiation. With better education and understanding of the anatomy of the region, a well-trained surgeon will spare the lymph nodes draining the arm, confining his dissection only to those which drain the breast, and the incidence of arm swelling should be minimal.

For eighty years after Halsted's first radical mastectomy, almost no change in the technique occurred, except for changes in incision, closure, and some modifications in wound care. Until recently, the basic tenets of the operation remained exactly as described by Halsted.

There are certain contraindications to the use of the radical mastectomy. The original contraindication primarily included those tumors that were beyond hope of cure — specifically, the inflammatory carcinomas and those which because of their size or deep involvement precluded reasonable hope of cure. Patients with such afflictions were in later years treated with radiation therapy, when this was available, or simple mastectomy (removal of the breast alone, sparing the pectoral muscles and axillary lymph nodes). While distant metastasis to liver, bone, or other vital organs was originally also a contraindication to radical mastectomy, in later years this contraindication was abandoned because it was felt that radical mastectomy provided the best prevention of local recurrence, which is the most dreaded nonlethal complication of the disease. A patient who might otherwise have lived a long and relatively normal life even in the presence of distant metastases may have her life made absolutely unbearable by the presence of local growth of the tumor in the skin and chest wall.

In Lucy's case, the tumor had spread to the axillary nodes, and since she later developed bony metastases in her neck, we know that the disease had already spread beyond the surgical area at the time of her mastectomy. The mastectomy still can be seen to have served its purpose, however, because despite her developing distant disease (controlled by oophor-ectomy and radiation) she never suffered the horrors of local skin recurrence. Lucy had radiation therapy at the time of her surgery because of the extensive spread to the lymph nodes. Had the tumor recurred locally at a later time, she would have been difficult to treat, since she had already received the maximum dose allowable to the skin in the area of her mastectomy. This type of recurrence is almost impos-sible to control by conventional means, even today, and therefore the radical mastectomy is still carried out, even as a palliative procedure in the presence of distant metastases.

Since we have just discussed practical examples of treat-ment based upon anatomic spread of the disease, this would be a good time to talk about actual staging as it is used today.

There are several different staging systems still in use, but they all attempt to categorize the degree of spread of the cancer and from that categorization to predict outcome on the basis of various treatments. No treatment studies can be compared unless there is agreement as to which stage each patient is in at the time of her treatment. Though there are differences among the several staging systems, these differ-ences are small, and the fine points are beyond the practical scope of this book. Basically, they all assess tumor size, lymph node spread, and distant spread.

Stage I includes patients who have small tumors (generally 1 inch or less in diameter), no lymph node spread, and no dis-tant spread. Simply put, this is *disease limited to the breast.*

Stage II includes patients who have slightly larger tumors, are positive for spread to the axillary nodes, and still show no distant metastases. In other words, this stage includes disease still in the early stages, but extending beyond the breast into the nodes.

Stage III includes patients with large tumors, generally posi-tive nodes, and no distant spread.

Stage IV includes all patients with distant metastases (for more detailed staging, see Appendix A).

It is important to note that we use *clinical* staging in assess-ing treatment, since that is all we have to go on at the time treatment is first decided upon and instituted. The *actual* stage may be different, but many years may elapse before the actual stage is known. For example, Lucy was a clinical Stage II, because she had a small tumor, positive nodes, but no diagnosable evidence of distant spread. However, she was an *actual* Stage IV, because the metastasis in her neck (found five years later) must have been present—though hidden—at the time of her original staging and mastectomy. The breast cancer had to have been present in her neck at that time even though it was not apparent.

Plus ça change, plus c'est la même chose

Jerome Urban developed what is known as the "super-radical mastectomy." Because there are some cases of spread to the lymph nodes beneath the sternum (breastbone), Dr. Urban hypothesized that patients with medial lesions (which spread to these internal mammary nodes) would not be cured by radical mastectomy and the axillary dissection. Dr. Urban introduced the dissection of the internal mammary chain of lymph nodes, necessitating the removal of parts of three or more ribs next to the breastbone and further dissection of lymph nodes beneath these ribs. This greatly increased the difficulty of the dissection and the morbidity of the procedure, as well as further deformity incurred by the permanent loss of the ribs in this area. Experience soon showed that this extensive surgery added little to survival, and the operation is rarely performed today. Furthermore, internal mammary node radiation adequately treats these nodes and the Urban super-radical mastectomy for medial lesions is therefore felt to be unnecessary by most surgeons.

The next step in the development of modern surgery for carcinoma of the breast became popular in the 1960s and 1970s with the introduction of the "modified radical mastectomy" (total mastectomy with axillary dissection). Today this comprises more than 80 percent of all operations carried out for carcinoma of the breast. It differs from the Halsted radical mastectomy in that the large pectoralis major and minor muscles are spared and, therefore, arm function is

largely preserved. In actuality it makes the operation somewhat more difficult, for these large muscles limit access to
axillary lymph nodes and the dissection is more difficult.
However, the cosmetic deformity is not nearly as great, and
a more normal-appearing chest wall and better arm function
can be maintained. The modified radical mastectomy stood
the test when compared with the classic Halsted radical
mastectomy and is now the mainstay of surgical treatment of
carcinoma of the breast. Newer treatments must now be
judged against this technique. The classic radical mastectomy
is generally reserved for tumors which invade the substance
of the pectoralis major muscle, a rare occurrence representing
late disease.

In the past few years, great attention has been focused on
doing less surgery for breast carcinomas. European physicians
pioneered this effort with surgery that consisted of wide *local*
excision of the cancer, followed by radiation to the breast.
The surgical rationale for continuing in the use of modified
or total mastectomy was based on the fact that for many
years it was felt that the more radical surgical procedures still
gave greater assurance of the prevention of the dreaded local
recurrence. In recent years, however, the development of
highly sophisticated radiation therapy techniques have once
again changed our views on the magnitude of surgical treatment required. It is true that radiation still has a certain destructive effect upon the breast and underlying chest wall.
However, cancer research is in a state of great flux at the moment, and more and more centers are investigating limited
surgical approaches followed by radiation in lieu of the
modified radical mastectomy.

The most recent approach to gain acceptance has been that
of limited segmental excision of the cancer and axillary
nodes followed by one of several forms of radiation therapy,
which will be discussed later. More and more evidence is
being amassed that points to the fact that local recurrence
after using this technique is about equal to that found after
the modified radical mastectomy. Radiation is an effective
method of treating axillary nodes, and the rationale for adding surgical removal of the nodes to the wide local excision

of the tumor is one of prognostication. Patients with positive nodes are more likely to also have distant spread, even if this is undetectable at the time of surgery, and are therefore candidates for chemotherapy.

It is unfortunately true that most surgeons are much more ready to regard the breasts of patients with cancer as expendable than are the patients. This view is not really derived from sexual chauvinism, but is rather largely due to a commitment to cure the patient at whatever cost. The chauvinism comes out later, however, in the tendency to regard the breast of a 25-year-old woman as sexually more important than that of the 50- or 60-year-old woman, when in fact women in the older age groups may feel as much or even more of an assault on their sexuality from the loss of a breast.

I was recently discussing the arguments for and against using limited excision and radiation as opposed to radical or modified radical mastectomy. A fellow surgeon listened to us for about ten minutes and I was appalled as he rose to leave and said, "I just don't see what all this fuss is about over a vestigial organ." Chauvinism is not yet dead. Preservation of a cosmetically and sexually acceptable breast should be available to all patients *if* it can possibly be done within the framework of a reasonable chance for cure and prevention of local recurrence.

When I first began writing this chapter, I was telling patients with breast cancer that I felt modified radical mastectomy still held the best hope for cure and prevention of local recurrence. If the patient had strong feelings about preserving the breast by using a lesser procedure, I would accede to her wish, adding a strong caveat about the increased risks she was taking. Some patients were willing to assume those risks.

Now that viewpoint has been completely reversed, and we apprise our patients of a newer concept, that "lumpectomy" (the medical term is *tylectomy*) combined with axillary node dissection and radiation seems to provide the same chance for preventing local recurrence, and the breast may be saved.

I now *suggest* the more limited resection, lymph node dissection, and radiation, but I will do a modified radical mastectomy if the patient feels more comfortable with the more classic approach to treatment. The caveat remains unchanged — only the emphasis has been reversed. Dogmatic stands on treatment are no longer acceptable, and today we are entering an era when the patient must be allowed in on the decisions of choice of treatment. Whether we call this "consumerism" or "informed consent" is a moot point. Either way, modalities of treatment are being reevaluated, and it is the responsibility of the physician to keep his personal prejudices under control in this particular area. Lucy was initially allowed very little leeway in her choices, and current surgical thought at that time allowed little choice. Today, however, I cannot dogmatically tell the patient that modified radical mastectomy is definitely superior to wide local excision and radiation therapy. The only certainty that I can foresee now is that treatment next year will very likely be different from treatment this year. Time may prove that very limited excisional biopsy followed by radiation is all that is necessary to assure reasonable hopes for cure. The ultimate goal, second only to prevention of the disease, would be to finally be able to follow John Hunter's suggestion that we abandon armed savagery for stratagem. That development is still beyond our horizons.

5

Did We
Get It All?

Lucy

"Damn. My neck hurts." I was playing tennis and every time I turned to hit a backhand a searing pain burned my neck.

I noticed it again that night when I was washing the dishes. "Must have slept on it wrong," I thought. When I lay down, the pain eased.

Four years had passed since my mastectomy. I was still being checked every three months by either the surgeon or the radiologist. Except for a lump in my breast, which had been aspirated and proven to be a cyst, I had had no complaints. I was healthy. Secretly, quietly, I thought myself cured. Some days I didn't even think of cancer at all. But one thing that is difficult to adjust to when you have had cancer is that you can simultaneously have an ordinary illness which is completely unrelated to that cancer. Each time I had a headache I wondered if I had a brain tumor. If I coughed, maybe it was in my lungs. Muscle aches became a reason for concern. I battled to avoid becoming a hypochondriac. I didn't like being so aware of my body. I felt betrayed by it. For so many years I had taken my good health for granted. I had observed the ritual of regular physical examinations. But I had never been sick. Now I saw myself invaded, abused, bereft. I felt raped. Still, I craved stability. And the only acceptable stability was good health. I felt well, therefore I was well. Except my neck hurt. It hurt when I stood. It hurt when I sat. It didn't hurt when I lay down. So I lay down as much as possible. I was worried.

At my next checkup with the radiologist, I mentioned it. Because I didn't want it to be important, I mentioned it casually. I told him I was afraid that I had bone metastasis, like an acquaintance whose breast cancer had spread to the bones and who now was terminally ill. "Don't be silly," the radiologist said. "You're not like your friend. She's had cancer all her life. You're different. You're all right." I liked that. I *was* different. I swallowed his assurances. I wanted to be well. I would be well.

And my neck continued to hurt. I didn't know how to judge pain. I had never had any. I was working, then, for a sculptor, as his business manager. But my neck hurt so badly I couldn't spend the necessary hours keeping his books. I was taking classical guitar lessons. My neck hurt so badly I couldn't practice. Driving became more and more difficult, so, when I decided to see an orthopedist, Betty took me. It wasn't time for my checkup with the surgeon. And hadn't the radiologist told me it was nothing to worry about? I wouldn't worry, but I had to find relief for the nagging, constant pain.

My regular bone man was out of town, so I agreed to see the young, new doctor in the office. He x-rayed my neck, and, finding nothing amiss, asked me where it hurt, when it hurt, how it hurt. All the while he was pushing, pulling, bending, probing. When he was through with the examination he pronounced confidently and sympathetically that I had a stiff neck. Butazolidin and four or five sessions in traction would take care of it. Sitting trussed and immobile in the traction device, I said to Betty, "I don't think he knows I have breast cancer and I just keep thinking there's a connection between the pain and the cancer." "Tell him," said Betty. "You tell him," I said. "I'm making a big deal over nothing and I'm embarrassed. Please. Just go mention it to him." If Betty did the talking then it wouldn't have so much importance. She would be protecting me. I wouldn't seem as concerned. So she went with the message and came back with the doctor. "Your pain has absolutely nothing to do with breast cancer. You have a stiff neck. Don't worry." So I tried. Not to worry. The prescribed traction made the ache worse, so I stopped after two sessions. But the Butazolidin alleviated the pain and I began to enjoy normal activity again, glad to be rid of the stiff neck.

It came back—my stiff neck. If I took the pills it sometimes quieted but I was aware of it even when it wasn't acute. When my appointment with the surgeon came due, I told him about my neck. "Sleep on a smaller pillow," was his advice. He was far more concerned with a small lump he had found in my breast. I couldn't feel it. He couldn't aspirate it so he sent me for a mammogram. It showed nothing. The surgeon was satisfied and I was dismissed — with a very stiff neck.

I had had reassurance from three different doctors. Two of them knew intimately that I had pre-existing cancer. Yet they denied that my bone pain necessitated any further examination. I should have been relieved. But I wasn't. I was, instead, very aware and very concerned. I felt foolish. Who was I to question their knowledge, their expertise? Yet I had done some reading. I knew that breast cancer, when it spread, metastasized to the brain, to the lungs, to the bones. The bones in my neck hurt. Was it metastasis? The doctors didn't seem worried. Should I be? I wanted to be well. Was I? They must be right. I must be wrong. And my neck still hurt. Had been hurting for more than six months — even though I slept on a small pillow. A tiny packet of fear lived with me.

When I called my internist to make an appointment for my yearly physical, I told his nurse that my neck hurt periodically and suggested that an x-ray might be in order. She agreed to pass the suggestion on to the doctor. Within hours she called me to say that the internist wanted bone scans done and that she had made the appointment.

It had been five years — that magic five years — since my mastectomy. Each New Year's Eve we celebrated. That was the anniversary date we chose, since I had found the lump on New Year's Eve. Often we didn't go to parties. Instead, we stayed home, privately, and toasted each other. We had made it one more year. We were alive and together. I was well. But, rather than being a joyous celebration, it was always tinged with a bit of sadness and a bit of fear. This year we had toyed with the idea of giving a party. Inviting all the doctors and saying, "Look. Five years. We beat it. We won the fight." But we didn't have the party. We pretended it was just another New Year's Eve. Not special or magic. And two months later I had an appointment for bone scans.

I didn't know what a bone scan was. Walking into the hospital's nuclear medicine department, I felt light-headed and sweaty. And even more frightened as I saw the signs on every door, warning, "Danger—radioactive material." A nurse gave me a shot in the vein of my arm. "What is that?" "Oh, just something to make your bones show up better." Wouldn't anyone ever give me credit for having a brain? For being an adult? For the fact that this was being done to me—and that I had a right to know what was happening? I asked again, "What is it that will make my bones show better? How does it work?" And finally she explained that the injected substance would circulate through my body and settle in any bone where there was activity. Activity? "What is activity?" But I knew. Activity was cancer. That's what they were looking for. Cancer. Again. Cancer.

The nurse told me that I could leave after the injection. It would take three hours for the radioactive serum to do its work. To settle. I had three hours to wait, three hours to think, three hours to fear. I didn't know then that after the three hours, the test itself would seem interminable.

The scanning machine had a cone which moved across my body, down a notch, and across my body again. There was an identical machine under the table, doing the same thing to my nether side. The length of the test was relative to the height of the person. I am very tall. So the testing took a very long time. Two hours. Two hours of no moving, no coughing, no scratching, no crying.

Journal Excerpt—March, 1975

The tests are over . . . I was at the hospital for six hours. I am exhausted and weepy and terribly fearful. . . . It was so much worse than I had believed. I am really as stricken today as I've ever been —completely irrational. Lying there for two hours, unable to move, unable to scream, unable to kick or hit or smash that machine ticking back and forth—saying cancer more cancer more cancer. It is so hard to describe the total fatigue and despair I feel. I guess pain would be worse. I'm pitying myself. I do feel sorry for me. I feel so sorry for me.

The nurse at the hospital told me that my doctor would give me the results of the scans. That meant two days of waiting. I hated to wait. I performed unconsciously, existing in a limbo.

The day before my physical, the doctor's nurse called again and told me to go back to the hospital and have a neck x-ray made. "Why can't I have it done at the office?" I asked. "The doctor wants it done at the hospital," she said. But she didn't need to explain. I understood. Five years ago I had a bone survey made at the hospital. The doctor wanted to compare the x-rays. I was more frightened. It was ridiculous to be frightened. Hadn't three doctors told me there was nothing to worry about? Why did I persist in being apprehensive? I could trust the doctors. They saw this kind of thing every day. Why shouldn't I believe them? I didn't believe them. I knew my body. I wasn't used to pain. I had had stiff necks before. I was desperately afraid that what I had was not a stiff neck.

My cousin Margaret called. She heard the fear in my voice. When I'm afraid, air rushes to escape through my words. I can't control it. I can protest and mouth my thoughts glibly enough, but there is always a telltale breathy quality in my voice. She offered to ride with me to the hospital and the doctor. I said no. I would go alone. She persisted. And I capitulated easily. I did need someone with me. Why had I pretended I wanted to be alone? Again, the role playing, the denial of my needs.

I had the x-ray and then went to the doctor's office. He told me quickly that the test results showed activity in my neck.

Shock and fear made me reel. The floor does fall away from your feet when you are shocked—and scared. I struggled to balance myself and hide my feelings. "So what do we do now?" (That should be the right attitude—undaunted, courageous, aggressive, positive.) I saw myself at a distance. I stood off to the side, watching some silly woman smilingly ask what to do when her neck showed a probable malignancy. My mind whirled with possibilities: They couldn't cut out the bad part of my neck because by head would fall off. What else was there? Now I would surely die. This was the moment I had dreaded. But the doctor was talking. What did he say? What did he want from me? What would he do to me?

He was confused. This wasn't his specialty, he said. He thought a biopsy ought to be done. He wasn't sure a biopsy could be done. It might be dangerous. I listened and watched and trembled. But I smiled. No tears. Don't cry. Don't let anyone know you are desolate. The office teemed with confusion. Calls were made. To the hospitals about the x-rays — they weren't ready. To the orthopedist for a conference — he wasn't in. I specified that the man I had seen six months before not be consulted. He hadn't listened to me. No one had listened to me. I didn't know anything. They were specialists. But they hadn't listened, hadn't cared, hadn't paid attention to Lucy. Dumb Lucy. Smart Lucy. Sick Lucy.

Margaret and I left the doctor's office. Nothing had been decided. But I had to get away from the people and the confusion. I promised to make an appointment with the orthopedist myself. We went to Margaret's house. My children were at home and I couldn't face them until I knew something more definite. I called Jack to tell him about the scans. He was quiet. He didn't need to talk. I could sense his awe. He said he'd come home early. Betty came over. She, Margaret, and I sat and looked at each other. Betty cried. I knew she needed to cry. Fear dried my tears. It made Betty's flow.

I called the radiologist. He was my friend. He would help me. He would know what should be done. He answered my questions easily. "Can that part of my neck be biopsied?" "Yes, of course. It's a very simple procedure." "Do you think it's cancer?" "Yes. I'm sure it is." "Then I am like my friend whose breast cancer metastasized to the bone?" "Yes. I'm afraid so." He was brutally honest. Yet I felt better after I talked to him. There was no indecision, no confusion, no evasion. Just truth. I could depend on him. Neither of us mentioned that six months before I had complained to him about my neck and he had pooh-poohed my fears.

When I got home the children had gone to their afternoon jobs. Jack wasn't home. I wandered around the house. I couldn't sit so I walked. And walked. And finally I made myself a drink—heavy on the scotch. I was walking and drinking when Jack got home. We didn't say much. He wept. He was lost and out of control. So I got stronger. I didn't need my drink. I only needed to comfort him. I promised him that I would do anything, go anywhere, see everyone until he was satisfied we had the best advice, the best treatment. We sat quietly then and loved one another.

Before calling the orthopedist, I called the surgeon and asked his advice about going to New York or Houston to have the biopsy done. He assured me that it was a very simple operation and could be done here. He said, "Don't worry." I was aware that everyone was telling me not to worry about myself. If I didn't worry, who would? And who should?

So the appointment was made. And we had two days to wait. Again wait. Worry and wait. We whiled away the hours running from one thing to another—a dinner party, a high school play, a fund-raising meeting. Anything. Anything to pass the time and to fill our heads. To help us forget what we were thinking about. We didn't talk about it to anyone. We spoke haltingly of it only to each other. Jack was, suddenly, irritatingly optimistic. Every time he voiced the possibility that everything would be all right, I got angrier. Why did he say that? Hadn't I told him what the radiologist had said? Didn't he believe him? Didn't he know? I knew. On one level I refused to be hopeful. On another I denied what was happening. My body had betrayed me again. Just when I had thought I was well, I had gotten sicker. Where was my control? Where was my will? What could I depend on? I floundered.

In the orthopedist's office, we looked at x-rays—x-rays taken two days ago, x-rays taken six months ago, x-rays taken five years ago. There were subtle changes in each picture. And now we saw that there was a hole in my neck. The bone was gone. Eaten away. No wonder it hurt. I insisted that the biopsy be done immediately. No, I didn't care if there was a private room. No, I couldn't wait any longer. I had to know. Now. So the operation was scheduled for the next day and I went home to pack my suitcase and check into the hospital.

Lying in the operating room, drugged but not asleep, my

main concern was the technique of cutting into the back of my neck. Would I lie on my stomach? Would I suffocate with my face crammed against the table? Would my hair have to be shaved off? What if the nerves in my spinal cord were damaged? I hadn't asked the questions before, so I asked them now. "I won't damage the nerves. I'll cut your hair very carefully. You will be sitting up when I operate." That made sense. If I sat up I could breathe. If I could breathe I would live. If I didn't have any more cancer.

I woke up in my room. I was sitting up with a brace, from chest to chin, supporting my neck. Someone told me that I had a metastasis. I don't remember who told me. It wasn't important. What mattered was that I was beaten. I had lost. There was breast tissue, malignant breast tissue, growing in my neck. That nauseated me. I felt dirty. I wanted to be free of my body. It was ugly, repugnant, hateful. Dying.

No one was very hopeful. The surgeon announced that as soon as I was stronger he would remove my ovaries. Estrogen is one of the hormones known to feed breast cancer and, since I was premenopausal, my ovaries still produced estrogen. No tests had been done to find if my cancer was hormone-fed. The test was available, but I was unaware of it. I agreed to have the operation. I didn't care. I had no fear of meno-pause. Wasn't it a natural phenomenon in the scheme of a woman's life? Anyway, what difference would my ovaries make? What difference did anything make? I was going to die. No one said so. I didn't ask. But I was very sad.

I cried a lot. I didn't mean to cry, but the tears came and kept coming. I was afraid. But the fear grew less acute. I felt very tired. Tired and sad, tired and sad and afraid. I lay against my pillows and smiled tired, sad, brave smiles. I spoke quietly to the nurses, thanking them for their kindnesses. I smiled sweetly at Jack when he came from the office. I smiled weakly at my friends and family. I wrote gracious thank-you notes for endless flowers and candy. I gave it all to the nurse's aides who brought me water and took my temperature.

I wasn't prepared for a metastasis. I had known it was a possibility — a probability. Yet I hadn't believed it. I was going to be different, I had always been different. Different was a good thing to be. But I had failed. I had fooled myself. The cancer had spread. I was the same as all those others — the others I had read about — the others I had seen at the radiation center — the ones who died.

A week later I had my ovaries removed. And suddenly people started talking about what to do next. I wasn't a part of the decision-making. I had been operated on twice in one week. I had learned that the cancer had spread to my bones. I was reeling, hurting, helpless. Forlorn. Doomed.

I listened to the doctors argue the options. Should I have more treatment? Should I go to New York for consultations? Should I see an oncologist? Had the cancer spread to other parts of my body?

Journal Excerpt — March, 1975

I know I can adjust to a reality. It is uncertainty that keeps me off balance. I have to wait for the cancer to catch a vital center, all the time listening to them say maybe we can stop it . . . maybe it won't . . . maybe maybe maybe. *How much easier it would seem from where I sit to know THIS IS WHAT WILL HAPPEN. I think I could be braver if I knew for sure. Jack says I'm not a coward. I wonder what his definition is — because I feel very cowardly.*

An oncologist was brought to my room, introduced, and we were left alone to talk. He was young and very earnest. His questions were forthright. How did I feel about having cancer? What did I hope for? What did I expect? I could only tell him that I wanted to live. I told him that Jack and I had celebrated our twentieth wedding anniversary and that I wanted to celebrate our twenty-fifth. He didn't answer. Only nodded. Then, "I'll help you however I can, but I won't be your shrink. You'll have to find someone else." It was my turn to nod. And I didn't tell him how frightened I was. That wouldn't fit the image I had to project: tough, realistic, controlled — the woman I wished I was! We ended our meeting as unaware of each other as if we had never met. He had seen a facade. I had seen another doctor.

He wanted me to go to Sloan-Kettering Cancer Center in New York City. He had trained there and wanted his teachers to consult with him on my projected treatment. Lung, liver, and brain scans were done; the appointment was confirmed; and, one week later, records in hand, Jack, my mother, and I left for New York. I had asked my mother to go with us. I thought she would be company and a comfort to Jack if I had to stay in the hospital for any length of time.

It seemed important to go to New York, to a big cancer center. The experts from out of town. It was, in fact, busy work. The examination at Sloan-Kettering was perfunctory, impersonal, not helpful. The doctor urged me to go back home. Do whatever my oncologist suggested. I have always suspected that it was only an exercise to build our confidence in my doctor. The trip caused no damage. But it was expensive and tension-ridden. It taught us nothing. Simply, it was a waste of time.

So we came home and settled down to live a normal life. Except that it wasn't normal. It was decided that no further treatment be given — except to wait and see if the hormone manipulation (the ovariectomy) would shrink the tumor. I had bone scans and neck x-rays every six weeks. A new spot showed up on the other side of my neck. I was frantic. The oncologist decided to wait still longer before starting treatment. A scan only shows activity. It can't discriminate between disease and healing. The new spot could be either one. He was very cautious. I was grateful for that. But I couldn't seem to stabilize myself. I quivered between doom and deliverance. Jack tried to be patient and understanding. I closed him out. And suffered alone. Miserably. He was confused and hurt. And angry.

Journal Excerpt — May, 1975

I have learned a good lesson. When I denied Jack the privilege of being my strength and comforter, I almost destroyed him . . . it was ugly and mean — the self-pity I have always tried to avoid. I will try not to do it any more. For if he is lost, there is no chance for me, and I know that now. I promise I will never again be that selfish. But I must have time for myself. I must be allowed that indulgence. Somehow we will work it out. He is so honest and good and I made him feel inadequate. Wrong. Wrong. How hard it is to live with this terrible thing.

Slowly I settled into a new routine. I was allowed no strenuous activity. So no tennis that summer. I felt sorry for myself about that. But I had never hated being alone. I read a lot, wrote a lot. I found a lovely, small meadow, completely surrounded by trees, hidden away, and I took a blanket and my radio and my journal and a book and spent hours there by myself.

I started working again for the sculptor. And I tried to sort out the thoughts that warred in my head. I couldn't stop thinking ahead. I was so afraid of what the next treatment might be. I wanted to know everything. Now. Where the cancer might spread next. When? What would the treatment be? How would that treatment make me feel? I had no pain at the moment. But the moment didn't concern me. I was afraid of tomorrow. And the more frightened I became, the more introspective and depressed I was.

Journal Excerpt — June, 1975

I always thought that if you could understand a problem, rationally carry it through your brain, give it objective alternatives, and come out the other side, you could lick it. But even though I can talk about it, and consider all options, I can't beat the depression. It's almost classical — staying in bed, avoiding contacts, not answering the phone. Jack is so patient. Unforcing but persevering — come on — get up — go with me — until I finally move. And even though I'm sad and quiet, it's better.

Suddenly I was menopausal. The idea hadn't frightened me. My mother had had a total hysterectomy at thirty-eight and, with artificial hormones, lived a normal, healthy life. She still was busy, involved, young-looking. She was my total experience with menopause. But I couldn't be given hormones. The whole point of removing my ovaries was to stop the estrogen activity. I wasn't like my mother. In the hospital, my internist had warned me of possible hot flashes and depression, caused by the ovariectomy. He prescribed Valium to counteract both symptoms. I had a hard time trying to decide whether the depression I felt was because I was menopausal or because I had metastasizing cancer. I concluded its source really wasn't important. But the hot flashes were another matter. They came with no warning. I learned to rip off scarves, unbutton buttons, roll up sleeves in seconds. I could handle the daytimes. But the nights were agonizing.

Journal Excerpt—July, 1975

I can't even lie down and rest without one of those goddamn hot flashes tearing through me—making me jump and turn into queasy dampness. I haven't slept well for nights. They wake me up like a leg cramp, making me tear out of bed and wait and wait until I stop being on fire. I want to throw things and hear them break. I am so tormented that I grind my teeth to nubs.

I began taking the Valium. Not during the day, only at night. And it helped. Every night I took 10 milligrams.

I started looking for books to read, books about breast cancer. I had been living in a vacuum of my own ignorance. Doctors told me what to do. I obeyed. It didn't help. I was getting sicker and I didn't understand what was happening. Feeling that the depression, the lack of control could be allayed by learning, I devoured every book, every newspaper, every periodical I could find. My library grew. My brain absorbed. Some of the information was misinformation. But I couldn't discern the difference. It was new. It was fascinating. It was depressing. But it was knowledge. I now had a platform from which to operate. If I had facts, even erroneous facts, then I could question. And if I could ask questions, I could learn. If I learned, I would have some control. There was still one unpleasant premise I had to accept: Ultimately, no one knew how to control breast cancer. It assumed its own growth, its own direction, its own timetable. I knew the only control I would have was the control of my treatment. To assume that control, I had to learn about all available treatment and what the manifestations of that treatment were.

Each new scan showed an additional spot — on my neck, my skull, my spine, my sternum. The oncologist kept saying, "Wait. Let's see. It might be a pre-existing lesion which is healing. Give your body time." While relieved that he indicated no further treatment, I lived with constant tension. If I put my hand to my neck, Jack immediately presumed I was in pain. He was always watching me. I was always watching myself. We maintained a stubborn anticipation of the next climax. Finally, miraculously, the scans became stable. They showed no new activity, and even a lessening of activity. The new spots indicated a healing process — not a growth of disease. The x-rays of my neck showed healing — the bone was healing.

The oncologist explained that this was what he had hoped for. He felt that the hormone manipulation was working. That there was a remission. I blessed my body. Finally, I had done something right. He also said that he felt the metastasis had been there for years. That the cancer had spread to the bone by the time I was operated on the first time. That made me very angry. All that time. Five years. Nothing done for five years while such ugliness was floating around in my body. Growing in my neck. The mastectomy. The radiation — was it all necessary if there were metastases already? Had there been scanners five years ago? In Louisville? In New York? Houston? Why hadn't I been advised? Could I trust a doctor again? They had treated me casually. Wasted time. Wasted my time. I had to seize control of my treatment. I had to learn about this damned disease. I would not allow anyone to treat me fortuitously ever again.

The radiologist and the oncologist had argued about treating my neck with radiation. The radiologist felt it should have been done immediately after surgery. The oncologist had wanted to wait. We waited. Now that he was sure a healing process was occurring, he gave the go-ahead for radiation. Radiation causes scar tissue to form, and the oncologist wanted to be sure he had a correct reading of the scans before he enacted any new procedure. I was scheduled for ten treatments. I didn't question the decision. The apparent fragility of my neck frightened me and radiation would give it strength. But it meant I would have to go back down into that hell — the radiation center — again.

Journal Excerpt — September, 1975

Tonight we went to Yom Kippur services — and I'll never go to temple again. That gobbledygook means shit to me. I thought I would scream. "Our father our king inscribe us in the book of life" — bah, humbug! What huge iniquity did I perform to get inscribed in the book of slow, tedious, tortuous death? My neck hurts. My throat hurts. I hurt all over. And what's more, I feel sorry for myself. So there. I'm angry. Jack wants to go with me to the radiation clinic tomorrow. I feel so mean I'd like to take him — and make him go downstairs with me into that horror and watch him cringe.

I did not feel euphoric any more. I knew that every three months there would be another scan. I lived in a three-month cycle. If I needed a haircut, I waited until after the scans. If I was due at the dentist, I made an appointment after my tests. I was afraid to plan ahead. I began living inside myself. I created a secret place. No one could touch me there. No one would know what I was thinking or how I felt. I indulged myself with pity. I was lonely but I was convinced that no one could understand my loneliness. Only I, who had cancer — great, growing cancer — could appreciate how it felt to be alive so tenuously.

Journal Excerpt — October, 1975

Jack talks about going away in February and it makes me feel sad. How can I get excited about February when my neck hurts today and God knows what tomorrow. I hate my life. I hate everything. And I don't want to think about trips and Christmas and birthdays. It makes me sadder.

We did take that vacation and I loved it. I was able to play tennis and ride horseback. I felt strong. But as soon as we came home I fell through the trapdoor of despondency. I waited for the tests. And when the reports were good, I exulted. Then sank back into despair. I was still reading everything I could find on breast cancer. I worried about the next kind of treatment. When would I need it? What would it be? What would it do to me? Discontented with today, I thought only of the future.

The oncologist was pleased that the hormone manipulation had been successful and that the remission was still in effect. Always concerned about what was to come, I asked what the treatment would be when metastasis recurred. Further hormone manipulation, he said. Since it had worked so well, he would either give me male hormones to repress the estrogen that the adrenal glands emitted or he would perform an adrenalectomy or hypophysectomy. I was horrified. And terrified. I knew that male hormones could cause hair growth, a beard, a deepening voice. I knew that an adrenalectomy resulted in dependence on synthetic chemicals. I knew that a hypophysectomy (the removal of the pituitary gland) was brain surgery and involved considerable risk. I had been wary when my neck was operated on. I couldn't imagine letting anyone near my brain.

No. None of that. I couldn't handle any of the treatments he mentioned. He had only discussed these alternatives in answer to my questions. No further treatment was indicated at that time. I was fine at the moment. But my mind flew off into the future.

Journal Excerpt—March, 1976

Can't seem to fight this one off. I'm lost—as if all will has been drained out of me and I just float along in total absence of reality. I'm so bitchy to Jack and he says, "Hey, why fight with me? I'm your best friend." He's right, but I'm better off alone. Then there's no need for effort. And no shame. Where's all that strength I was bragging about such a short time ago? I am completely victimized by my own damnable outlook, when actually I should be satisfied. Nothing has changed from the last tests.

Journal Excerpt — April, 1976

Last night I tried to tell Jack how lonely and despairing I felt and he got angry, and then felt full of guilt. I didn't mean to prompt either of those reactions. I only wanted to communicate to someone what was happening inside my head. I didn't mean that it was happening because of him or anyone else. I made a futile mistake and I mustn't make it again. Now I feel even lonelier. Jack says I should talk to a psychiatrist, but I don't want to. I know everything is my fault. I would love to go away all by myself. I'm so tired of trying. Nobody can understand. Jack and I used to be so honest with each other — now we seem to tread very carefully — making no waves. Who said no man is an island?

Journal Excerpt — May, 1976

I slept alone in the guest room last night. I can sense Jack's antipathy for me. And I really understand it. But I can't help it. I cannot rise above the creeping despair. I am thinking of taking those pills again — that's the first time in a long time. But I keep thinking of the children. And yet, the children's problems are too much for me to cope with. I can't or don't seem to care about anyone else. Just don't want to hear it — find it difficult to make casual conversation. Am not really happy alone — but certainly more comfortable. Jack and I seem to circle each other warily — it is strange and unlike us. I have lived a year too long. I haven't accomplished anything this year except to pull us all down into an abyss. Valiant is not an adjective for me.

Journal Excerpt — May, 1976

These last two days I have spent completely alone — thinking — really I don't know why I bother to get up and get dressed. The other night Jack made a passing remark — that he loved his car more than anything he's ever owned except me. And I got very angry — told him that in no way did he own me and never ever to think otherwise. But I keep thinking about it — and I don't think I own myself. If I did and was totally and solely in control of myself, I would kill myself. I suffer my indecisions in the light of my image reflecting off of the people who "own" me. And I realize it works the other way too — that parts of them are mine in return. When does suicide become so impelling that those interests become inconsequential? I want so not to be. If only the cancer would get out of my bones and into my liver or lungs. Or, better, if only I would just not wake up tomorrow.

Journal Excerpt — June, 1976

Robbie graduated from high school tonight. And as much as I have looked forward to it, I sit here alone, upstairs, while Jack is downstairs celebrating with all the kids. Here I am. I have to live and don't want to. Unless I take those pills. That's all I think about. Yet how to justify it to them? I can say what difference — I won't be here to suffer their hurt. But I can't get beyond that one yet.

I frightened myself. First I couldn't handle my physical ailments and now I couldn't manage my thoughts. When would total disability occur? When did I begin rationalizing my existence? I knew I had to do something while I still had some vestige of control. I needed help. Frantically, as Jack had urged me to do months earlier, I called my doctor and he referred me to a psychiatrist. I was ambivalent about talking to anyone. But the Seconal that I had stored and kept in a drawer by my bed was a constant fascination and, at the same time, an omnipresent danger. I needed help badly. Quickly. While I was still able to recognize my need.

I sat, uncomfortably, in the psychiatrist's office. Answering the academic questions he asked. Was I a moody person? Had I ever thought of suicide before? How long had I had cancer? When did it metastasize? What were the results of my latest tests? When I told him that the last tests showed remission, he asked the pertinent question — why now? Why was I so depressed now that I was better? I had no answer. "Think about it," he said. "We'll talk about it next time you come."

The question tormented me. Why now? Why was I so depressed now, when finally I had some time and some basis

for settling down? Time to get my bearings. Time to assess
the damage and establish a new philosophy for living. Instead,
I was using the time to destroy myself—or planning to
destroy myself. Why?

Just concentrating on the question seemed to slow me
down. The psychiatrist helped me realize that I had substi-
tuted the word "can't" for "won't." When I said, "I can't live
this way any longer," I was really saying that I wouldn't live.
That I didn't want to live. I could live. If I tried. If I wanted.
I was suddenly very conscious of how often I said, "I can't."
"I can't get excited." "Can't fight." "Can't understand."
"Can't care." "Can't handle." "Can't live."

I knew this was the most basic therapy—pages 1-10 of
Psychology 1. And it embarrassed me that I was so simple.
That the psychiatrist didn't have to read further than the first
chapter to help me. I preferred to think I was more complicated. Yet he did help me that easily. Of course, that I could
speak honestly, openly, without fear, of all the hopelessness
I felt was the real help. A finger on the button, the failsafe
button. I listened to him tell me not to assume a strength I
did not have. To stop protecting myself from my need for
comfort. He said, "Let Jack hear you cry. He won't mind. He
can help you." He warned that I had built my defenses so
tightly I denied myself room to move and change as events
warranted change. He assured me that my strengths and
resourcefulness had been eroded by real and stressful events
and urged me to be kinder and more patient with myself. He
told me that soldiers, on the battlefield, sustain such a high
level of fear that it cannot be endured. So they substitute
boredom. Tremendous heights of emotion cannot be sustained and that same letdown would happen to me, too. He
promised. And I believed him. I could believe him.

Depression wasn't put behind me quickly. But the decision
to see a psychiatrist was a crucial one. A wise one. He helped
me find a perspective to work with. He freed me of many
constrictions I had placed on myself. He taught me how to
ask for help and how to accept it. He showed me that it was
possible to regain control. And I needed, always needed, to
feel that I controlled what happened to me. I knew that I had

no control of the cancer. I had accepted that. But I must have control over how I lived with that cancer. I could manage my life. I had prepared myself for death. Now I would learn how to live.

I remembered my first meeting with the oncologist. I remembered his telling me he could not help me with any psychological problems. And I realized that no one, no doctor, had ever offered any help in that area. Surely they must realize that having cancer is more than a physical problem. Surely they must have had contact with depression over and over again. Yet they ignored its possibility. Even denied it. What did other women do? Were all doctors like mine? I had reacted so positively to such basic psychological therapy. I must have been unexceptional, within the realm of the expected. Why weren't my problems foreseen by the experts who were treating me? Was it possible that they didn't care? That it wasn't important to them? That life itself was all that mattered—not the modalities of life? I was angry. And my anger frustrated me. It accomplished nothing. I determined to channel it, to use the energy to educate myself. I would know so much that I would never, never be dependent on any doctor. Instead of a victim, I would be a partner in the decisions that affected my life.

While searching for information, I happened upon an article by Norman Cousins in the May 28, 1977 edition of *Saturday Review*. The article, "Anatomy of an Illness," had been reprinted from the *New England Journal of Medicine* and told the story of Cousins' own near-fatal illness in 1964. His disease was not cancer, but at the time he was given one chance in 500 for full recovery. These odds, curiously, did not stupefy him. Rather they energized him. He decided he had ". . . better be something more than a passive observer." I was fascinated. Here was a man who, when told he probably would never get well, said the hell with that! He actually refused to allow "the experts" to pass sentence on him. Cousins' doctor, too, was a most remarkable man. He was willing to cooperate with his patient, no matter how unusual the means Cousins employed. And Cousins believed that the ". . . full functioning of his endocrine system—in particular, the adrenal glands — was essential for combating . . . any ill-ness." He had read that adrenal exhaustion caused negative effects on body chemistry. He reasoned that if this were so, then wouldn't positive emotions cause positive chemical activity? And he formulated a bizarre course of action to test his theory. Most awesome was that this doctor agreed to his plans, cautioning him that while he had serious questions about it, he shared the ". . . excitement about the possibilities of recovery and liked the idea of a partnership." What a doctor. Nowhere in my relationships with doctors had I encountered such willingness to cooperate. Or even an indica-tion that I should have any input into the decisions about my treatment. I was overwhelmed. And envious.

Cousins explained that to exercise his positive emotions, he first had to get out of the hospital. His doctor agreed! So he moved from the hospital into a hotel room, with nurses, and he was immediately cheered by the lower costs, greater privacy, and the absence of unnecessary bed baths, linen changes, examinations by hospital interns. I nodded under-standingly as I read this. The next step was to stop taking the drugs prescribed for pain and sleep. He knew that these medicines taxed the adrenal glands. But he also knew ". . . that pain could be affected by attitudes . . ." and that he could ". . . stand pain so long as he knew that progress was being made in meeting the basic need . . ." of restoring the body's capacity to heal itself. Cousins felt that laughter was the most affirmative emotion. He had already called upon his own hope and faith. But there was nothing funny about the painful illness that kept him flat on his back. He decided that Allen Funt's *Candid Camera* films would be the answer to his need to laugh. And it worked. He found ten minutes of laughter gave him two hours of pain-free sleep. When he woke up, the nurse showed more films and he would sleep again. I could hardly believe what I was reading. Could it work? It seemed too simple. But it sounded so good, so possible. There were other unorthodox methods used, such as a slow-drip intravenous feeding of large amounts of ascorbic acid — and they all worked. He got well. Not overnight, but he was able to return to work and play tennis and ride a horse. It had been expected that he would never get out of bed. The experts had said so. But Norman Cousins proved them wrong. He said it was because ". . . the will to live is not a theoretical abstraction, but a physiologic reality with therapeutic characteristics."

Because he never accepted the prognosis, Cousins was never trapped in the fear and depression that accompanies an incurable illness. Would he have gotten well anyway? Was his combination of will and laughter and ascorbic acid just a series of exercises? Cousins shrugged the question off. He was willing to accept any and all criticism. He believed in the ". . . ability of the patient, properly motivated or stimulated, to participate actively in extraordinary reversals of disease and disability." He believed in ". . . the chemistry of the will to live." But he gave highest praise to his doctor,". . . who knew that his biggest job was to encourage to the fullest the patient's will to live and to mobilize all the natural resources of body and mind to combat disease." Cousins realized that his doctor's acceptance of him as a respected participator was the ultimate manifestation of the medical tenet, "Above all, do no harm."

I was elated by the article. It seemed to answer so many unformed questions, as if it had always been a part of my subconscious perception. I had been searching for so long for a tool to help me fight cancer. Suddenly I realized that the tool was me. I would help myself.

Journal Excerpt—October, 1977

This past month has been such a joyful one—so full of satisfaction and hope. The Norman Cousins article is always on my mind. I read and reread it—and I keep calling on my adrenal glands to help me. And they do. They are my god. It's important to believe in something—and so much easier for me if that something is within myself. Am I feeling too omnipotent? And am I using my adrenal glands theory as protection from the possibility that they might be removed? But I have felt it work. I have seen it work. I have called on them and they have responded.

I didn't tell anyone about my new philosophy. I hugged it to myself. It was too precious to put on display. And I, unlike Norman Cousins, was afraid that someone might denounce me; might call be foolish, or silly. But time made me more confident. My tests had been good for two years. I was alive. And I wanted to live. Any time I felt depressed, I exhorted my adrenal glands. If Jack and I had a fuss, I called on my adrenal glands. If the children argued or the washing machine broke, I urged my adrenal glands to work harder. Without being aware of it, I was practicing a kind of mind control. But what was most important was that I had a focus, a very positive focus, and it was working.

When I went for the next scheduled bone scan I was confident. Cocky. Feeling good. A little scared because the tests and the hospital always scared me. But hopeful. I knew I was fine. And I wanted the tests to prove it.

Damn. Damn damn damn. There was a new spot. On my scapula. I was shocked. How could it be so? I had no pain. I was discouraged. And disappointed. It was as if I were starting all over again. I wondered what I had really accomplished in the last three years. Yet, I felt my juices start flowing. I had been challenged. My right to exist was being questioned again. And I would answer. Yes. I would exist. I would live. On my terms, by my rules, but I would live.

This time the oncologist felt some action was indicated. He wanted to do a bone biopsy. He explained that while the growth was probably a metastasis, there was a chance that it was a false positive scan (a phenomenon that occurs for unknown reasons), and a far smaller possibility that it was a new, primary tumor. More scans were done for affirmation and—sure enough—the spot was there.

Eight years had passed since my mastectomy. I had lived with illness for eight years—illness, and fear, and loneliness. But I had changed. I had learned. And learning had given me strength. I could not accept blindly anymore. The oncologist had decided I should have a bone biopsy and, if a malignancy were found, radiation treatment. This time I would make my own decision. Never again would I listen and automatically obey. I knew where to get information. I knew what books to read. I knew which people to talk to. I would listen, I would study, I would question. And then I would determine, for myself, what to do.

The first person I called was my old friend, the person who

was always honest with me, the radiologist. He listened carefully to my description of the test results and the oncologist's plan. He disagreed. Explaining that he felt I couldn't have any more radiation to that area because of the extensive dose I had had after the mastectomy, he urged me to wait, to do nothing until I had symptoms—pain. He added that the scapula is an important bone and he objected to the risk of considerable discomfort and disability if it were damaged by biopsy. I wondered why the oncologist had suggested radiation if I had had too much already. Where were my records? Hadn't he read them? Or were they incomplete? I was glad I was involved.

But I now had two, conflicting opinions. What I needed was a third. So I called a cancer hotline. A woman answered. I gave her my medical history and told her of my quandary. She said she would consult a doctor and call me back. When she did, it was with the advice to have the biopsy.

Three opinions. Two to one. But I hadn't voted yet. And my vote was the crucial one. I weighed the differing judgments. The radiologist's reasons for no biopsy had been twofold: I had no pain, no symptoms; and I had had too much radiation already. The oncologist wanted to know what was going on in my shoulder bone. It could be a malignancy. It could be a false positive bone scan. He felt it was important to know. He and the orthopedist had assured me that the procedure was simple—that it held very little risk. And I knew of a new chemical that was being used to fight my kind of cancer. I knew what its side effects were. I was willing to try it if a malignancy were found. I needed to know. The reasons for biopsy seemed to outweigh the reasons for no biopsy. So my decision was to operate. And it was my decision. A small one—my first. I was proud of myself. I wasn't immobilized. I hadn't panicked. But I was scared and I wasn't optimistic.

Journal Excerpt—April, 1978

I'm back to ground zero—facing an operation again—that fucking hospital—how I quail at the thought. And then further treatment if it is malignant. With all the research and questioning and premature posturing, I'm still faced with an unknown. I wonder how important it is to try to know. With each phone call, each bit of information, I reel as if I'd been hit over the head.

The biopsy procedure was even simpler than had been expected. Much of the muscle in my shoulder had been destroyed by the radiation I had been given eight years before, so the orthopedist found an easy route to the bone. And I suffered little pain after the surgery. The orthopedist was pleased by what he saw. The bone looked clean to him. But the oncologist chaffed at our optimism. He warned us that our joy was premature. Bone pathology took three days, he told us. So we tried to quash our emotions. And wait. Keeping our feelings to ourselves. Fighting the pall that not knowing brought.

It was a very long three days, because it stretched over a weekend. And the oncologist, whose responsibility it was to get the report to us, didn't check with the hospital over the weekend. He took weekends off. We finally got the report ourselves. And it was good. So good. It had been a false positive scan. The spot had been nothing. The fault of the machine—a "false positive." Crazy term. It sounded contradictory. My bones were clear. No tumor, no spread. Not even a tiny bit of arthritis. How glad I was that I had had the operation. Now I knew. I knew I was okay, that I was still in remission. The hormone manipulation was still working. Never mind the hot flashes. Forget the depression. I was all right. My adrenal glands and I were effective. We were doing a good job.

My elation was shadowed by the anger I felt at the oncologist for not reporting the results as he should have. I found his casual attitude both thoughtless and unkind. So I wrote him the following letter.

Your delay in transmitting my pathology report created an unpleasant experience for all of us. But that is past. And the purpose of this letter is to try to establish a relationship or rapport that we can live and work with.

I should say to you, first, that I have the greatest respect for your professional ability, and feel quite fortunate that your services are available to me. Your advice, while sometimes differing with others, has been the right advice. You have been conservative in your treatment and I am grateful to you for that.

However, our relationship is one of interaction and, since it will be a relationship of some time, I would hope it might include mutual respect.

There is one most important need that must be satisfied to enable me to deal with having cancer. And that is the need to know. Not to know how long I'll live or how much I will suffer — you can't answer that — but to know what is happening right now, why it is happening, what should be done about it, and what results that treatment might have. In asking these questions I do not ever attribute you with omniscience. And I will continue to seek other opinions so that I may have the necessary satisfaction of making the final decisions about myself, for myself.

Included in my need to know is the need to know results of tests and procedures as quickly as possible. There is, for a family dealing with cancer, a constant sense of tension and a certain lack of spontaneity. We are learning to live with this. But when any testing is done — whether it's scans, x-rays, blood tests, or biopsies — the controls we exert are so taut, so heightened, that they leave us completely emotionless. It is an ugly existence. We can handle a good report and we can handle a bad report. The period of limbo is what we deplore. You said, once, to Jack, that I think I am special. True. And don't you feel you're special? And shouldn't each of us feel that way about ourselves?

I am fully aware that your interest in my cancer is only clinical. I accept the responsibility of all the rest. But you could make it so much easier by giving me the information I need freely, quickly, and graciously. It doesn't matter to me whether it's from you personally or referred to me by your nurse. If it disturbs you that I telephone, I'd be delighted to make an appointment and come to your office to talk — and pay you for your time.

Anger is an emotion that is unpleasant for me to deal with — not impossible, just unpleasant. And I would prefer feeling comfortable in the demands I make on you. I feel they are few but I sense that you feel otherwise.

Please communicate with me about this letter. That will be the first step. . . .

He did call me when he received my letter. And we did talk. I felt that we understood each other—at least on the subject of communication. It was a beginning. But I wondered if I would ever get over the feeling that all doctors are asses.

That beginning occurred eight years after I first knew I was sick. Perhaps I was a slow learner. Slow or not, I was learning. And my life reflected the satisfactions of that knowledge. I wasn't just learning about cancer. I was learning about living. And I was proud. I felt as if each day brought so many new accomplishments—on a very personal level. I wasn't changing the world. But my world changed constantly and it got better and better.

Journal Excerpt—September, 1979

Everyone has a momentous event in his or her life that changes his or her focus or direction. Mine is having cancer. But unlike a change of career, or marriage, or running for president, my big concern is something difficult to talk about. People don't want to hear. They're afraid—for me or for themselves. So I have to live quietly with the most important thing in my life—and I think I do it well. I've been creative, inquisitive, direct, and successful. But I still can't discuss openly, as others can, the central core of my life.

Tony

Lucy was led through a labyrinth of radiation therapy and hormone manipulation which was confusing and frightening. However, it was precisely these modalities of treatment which forced her metastases into temporary remission—and possibly even permanent remission. But Lucy was subjected to unnecessary fears purely because the element of the unknown was introduced. With a basic knowledge of both chemotherapy and radiation therapy as adjuncts to surgery, many of these fears could have been eliminated. While no one relishes the prospect of being treated for metastatic disease, a basic understanding of the principles involved will add tremendously to the patient's peace of mind and well-being.

Surgery and radiation therapy are directed at the primary tumor in the breast and at local involvement in the remainder of the affected breast and the lymph nodes.* Radiation therapy can also be directed at solitary distant spread, such as the bone metastasis in Lucy's neck. Chemotherapy and hormone manipulations are directed primarily at *distant* disease, whether in a gross localized area or in undetectable but *predicted* microscopic disease. Recalling the staging systems discussed earlier (p. 59), patients with Stage II disease have tumor *clinically* localized to the breast and axillary lymph nodes. However, as in Lucy's case, a significant number of these patients are actually in Stage IV (distant metastasis), possessing metastases which may not be detected with presently available methods. Thus, in turning to chemotherapy, we are treating distant metastatic spread, whether

*This chapter delves deeply into some rather technical medical points about chemotherapy, radiation, and hormone manipulation. Because critical decisions may be made on the basis of this knowledge, and because current practice is constantly changing, the reader is advised to discuss these choices with her physician.

diagnosed or predicted. When this treatment is started at the time of initial surgery it is called *adjuvant* chemotherapy.

Chemotherapy involves the use of various chemical agents which are eventually distributed via the bloodstream to treat distant spread. The major chemotherapeutic agents in use today act by interfering with cell metabolism. Some cancer cells multiply at a more rapid rate than normal cells, and these cancers will take up more of the poison than normal cells, allowing for selective killing by adjusting dosages. Furthermore, normal cells repair themselves more quickly than cancer cells and therefore can recover and repair themselves, whereas the cancer cells cannot. This same differential in recovery is exploited to kill cancer cells by radiation, as well.

The major chemotherapeutic agents in use today include cyclophosphamide, methotrexate, 5-fluorouracil, and Adriamycin. These drugs are most often used in combination programs known, respectively, as CMF (cyclophosphamide, methotrexate, 5-FU) and CAF (cyclophosphamide, Adriamycin, and 5-FU). The rationale for combining the drugs rather than using them singly is that each one attacks different chemical processes and in using a combination of several different drugs, lower dosages may effect a higher lethal action on the cancer cells. Some programs include two drugs in addition to the above-named ones: vincristine (a cell toxin) and prednisone, a drug similar in action to hydrocortisone.

WHO, WHAT, WHEN, AND HOW

In the past, patients who underwent mastectomy for carcinoma were not immediately treated with the chemotherapeutic agents. Rather, the physician waited for the appearance of gross metastases and distant spread before treatment was begun. However, Dr. Gianni Bonadonna of the Instituto Nazionale Tumori in Milan, Italy showed that adjuvant chemotherapy (chemotherapy begun at the time of surgery) was helpful in treating Stage II patients — those with spread to axillary nodes or beyond (remember that many of these patients, like Lucy, actually already have distant spread, even though it is not detectable). Dr. Bonadonna compared Stage II patients treated by radical mastectomy against those treated with mastectomy *and* CMF chemotherapy; after 27 months only 5 percent of patients treated with CMF had recurrence, while 24 percent of those treated with mastectomy alone had recurrence. Even with extensive node involvement only 9 percent of the CMF-treated patients had recurrence, compared with 41 percent of the mastectomy group. Long-term survival was 20 percent or better in the CMF patients. Postmenopausal patients did not do as well in this program as the premenopausal patients.

However, in a more recent study, 100 women who had four or more positive axillary nodes (found by mastectomy and axillary node dissection) were treated even more aggressively by adding vincristine and prednisone to the CMF regimen. This study showed even greater reduction in mortality and recurrence rates as well as a significant prolongation of the disease-free interval. Also important was the finding that postmenopausal women did as well as the premenopausal women — a sharp contrast to the Bonadonna study. The difference may be the result of adding vincristine and prednisone to the program, thus creating a more aggressive treatment regimen.

Since patients with positive nodes are more likely to have distant spread, even though this is not necessarily demonstrable, it is now felt that patients who have four or more positive lymph nodes at the time of surgery should be treated with the chemotherapeutic agents. The reason for choosing lymph node dissections even when radiation is used instead of modified radical mastectomy is that we still need to know the status of the axillary nodes so we can tell which patients will benefit from adjuvant therapy. Radiation is very effective in treating cancer in the axillary nodes, but only surgery will distinguish Stage I from Stage II patients (i.e., distinguish those who might benefit from therapy from those who might not). These programs of CMF, CAF, or either of these along with vincristine and prednisone are carried out with patients who have Stage II or more advanced disease for a period of about one year.

THE CHEMISTRY OF BEING A WOMAN

Many breast carcinomas are highly stimulated by the presence of estrogens. Therefore, it would seem that removal of the major source of estrogens, the ovaries, would benefit the breast cancer patient. This effect is most dramatic in the premenopausal patient who has high levels of circulating estrogens in her blood. However, it appears that removing the source of estrogens does not prolong total survival, although it does prolong the disease-free interval. It has been common practice until recently not to remove the ovaries until the patient develops a recurrence of the cancer. Those patients who then respond to ovariectomy (oophorectomy) prove their tumors to be estrogen-dependent and further hormone manipulations may be carried out for later recurrences.

The adrenal glands are also a source of some estrogen-like compounds, and after a period of response to oophorectomy, the tumor may again begin to get growth stimulation from the adrenal source of estrogens. In the past, when this occurred in a patient who had had a previous good result from oophorectomy, we had the choice of surgically removing the adrenals directly or indirectly blocking this estrogen production by removal of the pituitary gland in the brain (which stimulates adrenal function). Both of these are major operative procedures, involving significant risk and complications. They require that the patient take lifelong medication to replace other adrenal hormones. Clearly, this was not a procedure to be undertaken lightly, and it was reserved for patients who had had previous good results from oophorectomy.

Lucy had a long disease-free interval of five years (a good prognostic sign in itself, since patients with long disease-free intervals tend to respond well to chemotherapy and hormone manipulation) and her neck metastasis responded well to her oophorectomy. Now her next disease-free interval is almost six years, again a good sign. In the event that she develops another recurrence in the future, we would predict a good response to adrenalectomy or removal of her pituitary. But now there is even better news: She may not need either of those unpleasant procedures.

There is a substance within normal breast tissue known as *estrogen receptor protein*. This protein (ERP) can bind with estrogen in the cell and migrate to the cell's nucleus, where it has some effect upon the reproduction and multiplication function of the cells. Breast cancer cells may retain this receptor protein or they may lose the ability to produce it. Cancers which have estrogen receptor protein activity are called *ERP positive* and those which do not are *ERP negative* (this is determined by a now readily performed laboratory test done on the fresh cancer tissue taken at the time of biopsy or even from a distant metastasis).

Patients whose cancers are ERP positive are more likely to respond to hormone manipulation in the treatment of their cancers—e.g., oophorectomy, tamoxifen therapy, and even, in some cases, receiving estrogen. Whereas in past years we needed to see how a cancer responded to oophorectomy to know if it was hormone sensitive, today we can get a good clue by measuring estrogen receptor activity. Statistically, 80 percent of postmenopausal women will be ERP positive and 50 percent of premenopausal women will be ERP positive. However, since circulating estrogen levels are generally low in postmenopausal women, oophorectomy in these women is not often successful. In fact, some women's cancers actually regress following estrogen administration. The cancer too seems to have a certain ability to adapt its needs to a changing hormonal milieu.

The drug tamoxifen appears to act by binding to the estrogen receptor protein in the cancer cells and thus preventing the uptake of the actual estrogen, effecting what is called competitive inhibition. This means we no longer need to surgically remove the sources of estrogen, but can administer the tamoxifen instead. Thus far, tamoxifen has had an encouraging clinical trial. It will be several years before substantial statistics on its efficacy will be amassed, but the outlook is very promising.

In Stage IV disease 50 to 60 percent of patients respond to CMF or CAF (or CMFVP, CAFVP) programs; of those patients, 10 to 20 percent obtain complete remission while most of the remainder experience at least partial or temporary remission of their metastatic disease. This then becomes a very complicated area. There are many possible combinations not only of the types of drugs used but also in the timing in the use of these drugs. Statistics on survival and treatment failures are still being gathered in large numbers. Breast cancer (unlike other cancers, which are generally considered cured if there is no recurrence after five years) *can* recur after ten and even fifteen years. Long-term follow-ups of vast numbers of women are needed before we can determine a successful course of treatment.

Lucy's case illustrates this complexity very well. She underwent mastectomy at the time of her initial diagnosis and had twenty-three lymph nodes positive for tumor (near the maximum obtainable from the axillary dissection). This would put her in the category of the *premenopausal patient, Stage II*, with *probable* distant metastases. This prediction was later confirmed, since she developed biopsy-proven tumor in her neck five years later, making her *actually* Stage IV. At the time of her initial surgery, no estrogen receptor activity tests were available, so we do not know the state of her ERP at that time. Nor was adjuvant chemotherapy for clinical Stage II disease popular at that time. Lucy underwent local radiation in the form of external cobalt treatments totaling approximately 5000 rad. Her disease-free interval had extended to approximately five years when she developed a documented, biopsy-proven metastasis in the bones of her neck. At that time she underwent oophorectomy, and multiple bone surveys later showed that her metastases started to disappear. She then underwent local electron beam irradiation to the area to speed healing and has been free of disease for a subsequent six years. During that time she had what subsequently turned out to be a *false positive* x-ray suggesting tumor in her shoulder. This was followed clinically for a while and finally biopsied, but it was found to be normal bone tissue. She is, therefore, clinically disease-free and has had no further chemotherapy.

If she were to develop further evidence of disease, we would know that she was probably estrogen receptor positive, since she responded so well to oophorectomy. She would, therefore, be a very good candidate for tamoxifen and perhaps chemotherapy. If she were to have a solitary metastasis, we might merely treat that metastasis with tamoxifen and local radiation and await further development. If she were to develop more than one metastasis, we would assume multiple sites of tumor and then begin a course of chemotherapy. She would fall into the 50 to 60 percent response rate for at least partial response and have a 10 to 20 percent chance of complete remission as well.

We can see here that we are dealing with multiple modalities of treatment, possible for all stages of disease, and with possible long-term satisfactory quality of life even with proven Stage IV disease. Lucy Shapero has been alive and well and living in Louisville for ten years since her mastectomy. Thus, unlike other cancers, with which various modalities of treatment may be ineffective, breast cancers have a wide biologic spectrum and are readily treated with multiple forms of therapy.

YOU'RE NOT GOING TO POISON ME!

There are many myths and old wives' tales regarding some of the side effects of chemotherapy, and the initial reaction of most patients is to refuse treatments. The most commonly mentioned effect is hair loss, which does occur. However, this is temporary and the patient generally regains normal and even improved hair growth following the discontinuance of chemotherapy. Some patients have nausea and vomiting, but this is temporary and treatable. The most significant problem is what is known as granulocytopenia, the reduction in the manufacture of white blood cells by the patient's bone marrow. This is a significant problem, because when the white blood cell count goes below a certain level, the patient is very susceptible to infections. Generally, this is an indication for temporarily stopping treatment and allowing the white cells to return to normal.

The biologic activity of breast cancers is so variable that the breast cancers seem to adapt to treatments over a period of time and may become, for example, resistant to estrogen withdrawal and in some cases may regress following the administration of estrogens — quite the opposite of the initial characteristics.

There are still two characteristics of breast cancer which make it different from most other cancers. The first is the question of the long latent periods between the onset of disease and emergence of the metastasis. We have no idea what it is that keeps the cancer cells alive but dormant for as long as 15 to 20 years and then triggers renewed growth after so long a quiet period. It may have something to do with the biochemical and hormonal milieu in which the cancer exists, or more likely may be something in the natural host defenses that the patient uses to keep the cancer in check until it escapes this control. These are still very uncertain areas for us today; and equally as uncertain is the question of *biologic predeterminism*.

THE INEVITABLE

Some scientists feel that the die is cast from the moment the diagnosis of cancer is made, and that we only manipulate the disease, and do not alter the time and mode of death. Though the theory of biologic predeterminism is still in large part unproven and does find support in some of the more aggressively lethal cancers, the situation is not so clear-cut in breast cancer. Even if the die is indeed cast at the time of diagnosis, we still exert strong influence upon the time, course, and quality of life with the weapons at hand today. Surgery, radiation, hormone manipulation, and chemotherapy have all expanded geometrically in recent years, and the multidisciplinary approach to the disease has had profound influence on the quality of life for myriads of women.

The final weapon in our armamentarium is an old standby which has expanded rapidly with the new technology of today: radiation therapy.

RADIATION THERAPY

The popularity of radiation therapy has gone through several cycles since its inception. Initially it was used as an adjunct to treat the mastectomy site and regional lymph nodes. Later, as chemotherapy expanded and became a useful alternative, radiation took a secondary role. Now, with the advent of newer technology and the increasing demand of women to try to save the breast while curing the cancer, radiation has resurfaced in both primary and secondary treatment.

As with chemotherapy, this is a highly technical subject, and a minicourse in nuclear physics is in order — there will be no final exam.

Though shrouded in mystery and space age technology, radiation is merely one more use of energy, similar to the energy used in more familiar applications, such as heat or light. Just as the kinetic energy (that of movement) of a bullet can be converted into heat energy (when slamming into a target) and thereby cause some destruction as the energy is released, so can radiant energy be aimed and converted into one form or another of destructive power. The analogy holds true for the force of radiant energy as well: Both bullets and radiation tend to be more destructive as their energy of origin increases (most of these radiation particles travel at nearly the speed of light).

The sources of this radiant energy are the very tiny particles which make up the atom. The simplest way to describe an atom is to liken it to our solar system, with the nucleus of the atom representing the sun and the orbiting electrons representing the planets. This, of course, is a slight oversimplification. These tiny particles (invisible to the most powerful microscope) have electrical charges — the nuclear protons are positively charged and the electrons are negatively charged. Thus by using magnetic equipment these charged particles can be accelerated and directed to specific targets—in this case, the cancer.

There are several types of atoms which are inherently unstable, and it is their nature to release some of these charged particles at high speeds. We take advantage of these high-speed charged particles by using them as our "bullets" or sources of energy. Just as light can penetrate solid glass, so can these tiny charged "bullets" penetrate human tissue and release energy capable of destroying what cells they may strike. If we can direct them to the cancer cells, they are capable of destroying these cells, but may also destroy any normal cells they strike en route. Just as chemotherapy can be manipulated to do *more* damage to the cancer, so can radiation be manipulated to selectively destroy cancer cells. The major advantage of chemotherapy is that it can be distributed diffusely throughout the body to destroy small, invisible cancer metastases, while a "visible" target must be available at which to aim our radiation "bullet."

There are two basic sources of these radiation bullets: radioactive atoms, such as cobalt-60, cesium-137, and iridium-192 (the number describes the atomic weight of the atom), and electromagnetic energy derived from the orbiting electrons themselves. The electromagnetic energy is similar to that used in the common diagnostic x-ray machines, but with much higher voltages and therefore higher destructive energies.

The radiations of cobalt, cesium, and iridium are released directly from the elements themselves and are directed to the patient by opening a window in the shielding machinery, much the way a camera shutter opens to let in light.

Electron beam therapy utilizes a machine called the linear accelerator (LINAC), which uses a magnetic field to accelerate electrons to high speeds and then fire them at the target. The target is the cancer. One might visualize this as a hammer striking an anvil and releasing a spark: The hammer is the high speed electron striking the cancer (the anvil) and releasing electromagnetic energy (the spark). It is this "spark" of energy that kills the cells.

Finally, we measure the doses of energy delivered, and express these dosages in units called a "rad." There has recently been a change in terminology to a system of "gray." One gray — named for the English physicist Lord Gray, who developed dose measurement in radiation — equals 100 rad. To give you an idea of the relative energies involved, an ordinary chest x-ray delivers a very low amount of radiation, about 0.02 rad, while low-dose mammograms yield approximately 0.03 to 0.05 rad. By contrast, the usual total dose of radiation delivered to the breast is about 5000 rad of energy, with a booster dose of an additional 2000 rad when iridium is implanted near the cancer site itself.

Cobalt therapy has certain limitations, despite the fact that the equipment involved is relatively simple to use and cheaper to run than the linear accelerator. Technically one has only to open and close the "shutter" and allow the radiation to strike the target, the dosage being regulated by distance from the target and time of exposure. However, the energy output is fixed at about 1.25 million volts; by contrast the linear accelerators can deliver 10 million volts or more.

The linear accelerator has some advantages over the more conventional cobalt units. The advantage primarily concerns what is known as the penumbra, or shadow. Linear accelerators can deliver their radiation to a field with an incredibly sharp border, so that no scatter of rays (penumbra) occurs outside the edges of that predetermined field. Cobalt cannot be controlled sufficiently to eliminate the area of penumbra. Furthermore, the biophysics involved in release of the higher energies delivered by the LINAC allow better penetration in depth to the cancer and less irradiation of the skin.

Iridium has its own advantage. Since closely grouped sources are used in the implant, there is a distribution in the neighborhood of only 1 inch. Thus, if inserted near the cancer, the iridium irradiates only very small amounts of tissue, sparing the surrounding normal cells (for example, those of the lung).

From a practical viewpoint, how do we use these different sources of radiation to treat breast cancer?

Cobalt has been the mainstay of radiation therapy for many years, but it has the disadvantages of lack of sharp margination and lower fixed energy output. The advent of linear accelerator therapy has enabled us to deliver higher energy to discrete tumor targets and thus better spare the surrounding normal tissue. The accuracy of the LINAC x-ray beam is extraordinary—very large dosages of energy can be accurately delivered to a precisely defined area.

Today, programs of irradiation can be carried out in several ways. When "lumpectomy" is the sole surgical treatment, the breast is irradiated with cobalt or LINAC-generated x-rays to 4000 to 5000 rad to destroy any residual cancer cells which might remain, as well as any other foci of cancer within that breast. The x-rays may also be used to treat the axillary and internal mammary nodes if these are not surgically removed.

Iridium comes into play in treating the local area close to the site of the primary cancer, especially if it is felt that any gross tumor remains or surgical margins are too close to the cancer. Using light general anesthesia, small polyethylene tubes are inserted in a gridwork surrounding the cancer site. Then small iridium wires encased in plastic are inserted into the polyethylene tubes and allowed to remain in place for 36 to 60 hours, depending on the dose desired (usually an additional 2000 rad over and above the 5000 rad delivered to the whole breast by the cobalt or x-ray treatment). During this time the patient is fully ambulatory and requires little if any pain medication. Then the tubes containing the iridium are removed by merely pulling them out, without the necessity of any further anesthesia.

Finally, distant metastases—in bone, brain, or liver, for example—can be targeted by conventional x-ray techniques and/or synchronized with electron beam therapy, as was the case with Lucy's neck metastasis.

Irradiation is usually begun as soon as wound healing from the primary surgery is complete (four to six weeks) and is carried on on an outpatient basis.

The 4000 to 5000 rad of radiation administered to the whole breast is usually delivered in small divided doses, five days per week for four to five weeks. There are two reasons for the small, divided doses. First, cancer cells are most susceptible to radiation kill (or destruction by chemotherapeutic agents) during two phases of their growth: when they are manufacturing DNA (the chemical of reproduction) and during cell multiplication. By dividing the doses and eliminating two days a week, the probability of striking the cancer cell during these specific phases increases. Second, normal cells recover from radiation better than cancer cells, so by dividing the doses, we give the normal cells a chance to recover before the cancer can "catch its breath"; thus high cancer-killing doses can be given.

There are very few side effects of administration of radiation to the breast and lymph nodes, unlike irradiation of, for example, the stomach, which occasionally causes nausea and vomiting. In addition, accurate targeting avoids irradiation of the lung.

Radiation does affect the skin, and patients may get temporary redness and swelling much like a severe sunburn. This is not actually a "burn," in that heat is not the cause of the redness. Radiation dilates the small blood vessels, which accounts for the appearance of a "burn," which is of short duration and rarely causes any serious problem. The irradiated breast does tend to become firmer with the passage of time, but cosmetic results are excellent, certainly superior to those with any mastectomy.

There has been a great deal of talk about the possibility of radiation being a *cause* of some forms of cancer, which indeed it can be (witness the Hiroshima experience). However, diagnostic levels such as those used in low-dose mammography (0.03 to 0.05 rad) are extremely low, and the benefits of detecting early curable cancers far outweigh any theoretical risks. The higher doses used years ago to treat acne and thymus tissue in children did indeed cause an increase in cancers (skin and thyroid cancers), but these techniques have long since been abandoned. Very high-dose radiation used in breast cancer has not proved carcinogenic.

The technique of lumpectomy, axillary node dissection,* and whole breast irradiation has been used for many years in Europe and Canada. Recent studies by Dr. Samuel Hellman at Harvard have provided very encouraging results. Thus far, results of this treatment are entirely comparable to results achieved with the more classic modified radical mastectomy. Hellman's studies extended to five-year follow-up, while those in Europe and Canada extended even longer. It is significant that much of the impetus for the adoption of this type of therapy came from women who refused to be forced into the classic treatment and insisted on their breasts being saved.

Recent studies from the Curie Institute in Paris have substantiated Hellman's studies, as well as those done earlier in Europe and Canada.

HAVE IT YOUR WAY

Once again, we should recall that there is today no place for dogma in the treatment of cancer. Techniques are changing too rapidly and the statistics are too variable for us to deny any patient access to any one of several modalities. Treatment is a multidisciplinary program and no *single* therapy is sufficient to provide the patient with adequate chance for cure. The team approach, while having some drawbacks (as Lucy has seen in the disagreements among her physicians), is still the approach that will give each patient the highest chance of survival.

If, indeed, the biologic die is cast when we first see the patient, we still have a multiplicity of effective weapons, so that when the cancer escapes one modality we can turn to another. Radiation doses are finite, and once total tissue dose

---

*Since Stage I cancers (those without lymph node metastases) are not treated with chemotherapy, and Stage II cancers (those with lymph node metastases) may be treated with chemotherapy, the status of the axillary lymph nodes is still important.

reaches maximum, no further radiation treatment can be given for the duration of the patient's life.

YOU'VE COME A LONG WAY, BABY

At the present time, there is no clear-cut answer as to whether radical surgery or limited surgery augmented by radiation is the best mode of therapy. However, if present studies stand the test of time, we can expect to see a gradual shift away from the classic surgical precepts and a shift toward more limited surgery for diagnosis and prognostic lymph node biopsies, followed by local whole breast radiation. If this is indeed the case, as present studies suggest, we have come a long way from the classic Halstedian dogma of ninety years ago.

6

What Do I Say to Them Now?

Lucy

Ten years ago, when I found the lump in my breast, I went alone to see the surgeon. Jack stayed home to baby-sit. He had offered to go with me but I insisted I could manage by myself. I was frightened of the possibilities. But they were merely possibilities and until I knew otherwise, I would prove my courage by showing independence.

Examining my breasts, the surgeon glanced at me and said, "Hey hon, calm down. You're hysterical." And I seethed with anger. Why had he said that? I hadn't uttered a word. There had been no tears. I didn't want him to think I was hysterical. Hadn't I come, wisely and alone, to be checked? Certainly I was worried. I had a lump in my breast. But hysterical? No.

His accusation contributed to the tenor of our relationship. He had presupposed that, faced with the probability of cancer, I would be hysterical. I wonder now if perhaps he, faced with cancer, would be hysterical. But it is dangerous to ascribe imagined emotions to other people. It stunts relationships. However, I often had to struggle to understand my doctors in order to realize why they did not understand me.

Part of the anger I leveled at the surgeon was misdirected. True, I wasn't raving or wild or weeping. But I was frightened. And it probably showed. He had merely chosen his words badly. I might have changed the course of our relationship if I had said what I thought: "Don't tell me how I feel. Don't ever assume you can know what I'm thinking. I'm not like everybody else. If you want to know how I feel, ask me. Or listen to me. Don't ever presume." But I said nothing. And our communication has been precarious ever since.

After the mastectomy I was hesitant to ask many questions of him. He seemed to push my emotional levels up a notch. When I thought I was calm, he thought I was agitated. When I was dejected, when he told me of the lymphatic spread, he assumed I was desperate. It was easier to limit our conversations. He didn't seem comfortable dealing with feelings. And he made me feel uncomfortable with my own.

So I had to look further for someone to talk to. I needed someone with professional knowledge — an authority. And I found the radiologist. When he came to my room to talk about the proposed cobalt treatment, he was a stranger. When he left, I had an ally who would share my ordeal. He was relaxed, with no apparent restrictions on his time. If I was serious, his answers reflected my seriousness. If I cracked a joke, he laughed and bantered with me. It was important to feel we could still laugh. He listened and heard what I was saying. When we were through talking, he knew who Lucy was. And I had a friend, a knowledgeable friend whom I could trust and question and depend on. It didn't take a great amount of time — maybe forty-five minutes. But that forty-five minutes proved the most valuable of our association.

He was no more dedicated to his work than was the surgeon. Nor was he more skilled. But he realized the value, for both patient and doctor, that listening can give to a relationship. We didn't always agree, yet he never ridiculed my ideas. He was sympathetic, interested, and caring. I have shared my entire cancer experience with him and whether or not we agreed on the proposed treatment or current philosophy, he has always been supportive. What luck to find a professional who cares so deeply for his patients' quality of life.

I had refused help from Reach to Recovery. I was afraid that help would reduce me to a small member of a large group and I couldn't stand being placed involuntarily into a club that I hadn't chosen — whose members I didn't know. Where the only common link was one breast less than normal. But support from Reach to Recovery might have given me answers I needed. If I hadn't been so stubborn, I might not have had to search for an individual to give me information.

The inherent drama of the words "you have cancer" packed such a wallop that I reacted instinctively, rather than calmly sitting down and formulating a method of behavior. A lack of thought for others, a visceral, mindless impulse, made me talk openly about my illness. And it became my charge to direct the kinds of talk and emotion related to it. Before I knew how I felt, I attempted to bend the way others felt about me.

I had always been a talker. I knew intuitively the only way I could handle having cancer was to be open about it. How could I live with one breast and pretend I was the same person? How could I exist with the real threat of death and pretend I didn't feel that fear? How could I continue having open and honest relationships with people if I hid the most consequential part of my life?

It is reasonable, is it not, for a mother, watching her older daughter suffer with cancer, to wish it were she who had the pain instead? And is it credible for a husband, told that his wife has cancer, to fight the fear of her death and his own loneliness? To cling to hope, tenuously? Would it be justifiable for the children of that daughter and wife to hear the truth about their mother, and then to tuck that hateful truth deep down into their souls, never mentioning it aloud? As if nothing had changed?

I watched my family react this way and I understood. I saw the aching in my mother's eyes. I watched Jack's face. Saw the muscle twitch as he resolutely held my hand and watched me cry. I listened to the children recount the daily sameness of their school activities. I heard them plan outrageous parties and nag about restrictions. But I refused to allow them to manipulate me into corners I hadn't chosen.

I needed my family. And they rallied around me so strongly I never considered that I might be forcing them to deal with my illness only on my terms. They accepted my direction, encircling me with their love and protection.

I didn't want to be alone. There was too much to think about and too much to be afraid of. Yet I didn't want my friends to see me cry. I was still too concerned about my image. I couldn't allow them to see the rawness of my spirit until I had some control. So my family became the buffer between me and the existence I tried to assume. I could trust them because they loved me whether I was cheerful or bitter. They would accept me whether I was whole or maimed.

We told the children the truth: I had cancer, my breast had been removed, and I would get well. They accepted what they were told, and, as our lives resumed a normalcy, seemed to put it behind them. After all, within months I looked the same, took care of them as always, continued working and playing as I had before the operation.

Shortly after I came home from the hospital, Robbie, our then eleven-year-old, asked me for money to send flowers to a school friend whose father had died of cancer. I asked who it was and was stunned to find that I knew him. How could he have died a week before and I not know about it? I confronted Jack and he explained that the man had kept his illness a secret. Okay, but why wasn't I told of his death? Why hadn't Jack told me? Why hadn't Betty, Dann, someone told me? And I realized I was being protected from such grim realities. I guessed it was assumed if I weren't told that people died of cancer, then I wouldn't think I might die of cancer. It was a stupid supposition and I was inordinately angry. When I calmed down, Jack promised he would never attempt to protect me from the truth again.

But my friend had concealed his illness from his children. And I worried that I had made a mistake by telling ours the truth. They were so young. Could they handle the pain of knowing their mother had cancer? Was I selfish to demand such openness? I worried that I had been too hasty, not considering the ramifications before I talked so freely. I was doing things my way, but now I felt the first painful twinges of guilt.

I knew my family needed certain reassurances from me. They needed to know I would get well. They needed to know I wanted to live. And they wanted to feel everything would be the same as it had been before. But I wasn't sure I could give them what they needed. Still, I needed them to protect me from my doubts. We struggled to accommodate each other.

My sister Betty, my brother Dann, and I had always been

close. We had never examined our relationships. We were
children of the same parents. We loved each other. And that
was just how it was. But with my illness as a catalyst, the
surface began to ripple.

Dann came to see me every day while I was in the hospital,
and afterward when I was recuperating at home. Our visits
were pleasant. I was always glad to see him, aware of the time
he shared with me. But one day, when he came, I began to
tell him of my growing depression. He interrupted me, saying, "You'll be over it soon. Everyone gets down now and
then." He made it clear that no ugliness should intrude on his
visit. He didn't want to know. He loved me. Didn't he show
his caring by visiting regularly? But those visits were to be
happy times. And I accepted his unspoken rules.

My relationship with Betty was different. Rather, Betty
bled when I hurt. And I often felt guilty because I always
told her when I hurt. She made time, no matter what her
other responsibilities, to drive me to the radiation center,
to come for lunch, to listen to me feel sorry for myself. I
eagerly accepted her attentions and her tenderness. But I did
feel guilty because she gave to me unstintingly and I eagerly
took as much as she could give. I tried sneaking to the hospital for tests so she wouldn't feel she had to go. But that made
her unhappy. And I realized she needed to be attentive, and
if I needed her — well, then — that was fine.

When I was first diagnosed, Betty called Tony, her brother-
in-law, my co-author, for information and for, hopefully,
solace. Tony gave her all that she asked, but he also realized
Betty's inherent danger. After all, she was my sister, my
mother's daughter, niece of my aunt. The incidence of breast
cancer in our family was horrendous. And now, with my
diagnosis, the odds were stacked against her. Tony was certain her chances of having breast cancer were appallingly
high. To quiet him, Betty promised to have her breasts examined every three months.

Often we went to the doctor together — I had to be
checked too — and we would sit in the waiting room, breath-
less and sweaty, making bad jokes to keep our spirits high,

waiting to hear if we had a reprieve until the next three-month examination. How could we have been closer? We had the same hopes, the same fears—for ourselves and for each other.

Betty had a cystic condition and worried about the constantly changing lumps and bumps. When a biopsy was indicated, we held our breath until the lump proved to be only a cyst. Relief. Great, joyous, welcome relief. But temporary. There were always cysts and the concern was ever-pressing. She struggled to live without fear. I watched her and felt guilty. My cancer had brought this hellish stress into her life. And it wouldn't go away. Ever.

My family gave me protection and care. And so did my friends. Overwhelmingly there was love, yet I posed a threat to many of them. The word "cancer" is formidable. The idea of cancer so terrifying. It is like death—we try not to think about it, hoping it will go away. Yet I was here. I didn't go away. And my friends reacted in different ways. Some listened to what I had to say. And answered what I said. Some pretended nothing had happened. Some assured me everything would be fine. And others stayed away.

Perhaps I was cruel to those who, in any way, denied my truth. I demanded that they let me operate openly. I refused their platitudes. I ignored their aversion. And the friends I loved, loved me enough to try to see my illness through my eyes. Oh, sometimes they cringed at my black humor. And sometimes they wept when I spoke despairingly of my future. But they kept trying. They were, indeed, friends.

Only Jack wholly allowed my stumbling, anxious, fearful attempts to reestablish my identity. To fight through the pain and fear and isolation. He was the person who, when I cried, said, "I don't blame you." Who listened and listened and listened while I endlessly repeated my feelings of self-pity, loss of control, anger. I saw his sorrow as I ranted about dying. But he listened. And he said, "I understand." He allowed me the time, alone, to think—never demanding to know what I thought. Never lecturing, but always ready to hear and comment. He was not only a comforter. He was a confidant. And the bond between us strengthened.

Some women wonder if their marriages will withstand

breast cancer. I found myself wondering if we would have had such a relationship if I hadn't gotten sick. Jack revealed an empathy I hadn't known he had. Never did I feel unwanted or misunderstood. He seemed to sense what I needed, when I needed it. And I stretched to anticipate him in the same way. As more and more of our friends separated and divorced, I found myself aware that I was grateful to my illness. I knew that it forced a new dimension on our relationship. We knew how much we needed each other. And, ironically, we felt very lucky.

When the cancer metastasized and I realized that all of my doctors had missed the diagnosis, I again went through a period of anger and resentment. The knowledge I had gleaned hadn't been great enough to participate in my diagnosis, and I hadn't been able to depend on any of the professionals. I tried to understand the doctors. But all I could feel was a tremendous sense of isolation. I never talked to them about it. It bewildered me to find them so careless. My respect for them was greatly diminished. I had wanted them to be all-knowing, all-caring, wise men. But their feet were mired in clay. And, still, I had to deal with them. No matter that I now questioned their omniscience — my life depended on their skills. I would have to learn an important lesson: to forgive what had already happened. There was nothing anyone could do about what was past. What was important was the present and the future. I must know what was happening — and what might happen. Doctors generally don't like to be questioned. They don't like to speak to possibilities. Never again could I totally trust a doctor with my life. I would have to learn more about my illness. I would have to find resources I could depend on. My bitterness and anger quieted. I had expected too much. Doctors are not artists. They are not gods. They are technicians. And sometimes they make mistakes. The more knowledge I have about my body-machine, the better I can help my doctor repair it.

The metastasis created fear, too, for our children. They were five years older — much more aware. And I was glad that I had been honest with them. For, as I gave them the facts — that what had happened wasn't good but I wasn't going to die; that the treatment would give me time and then I would have more treatment—they considered what they heard, knew that I had never lied, and believed what I said.

One night, after receiving a particularly discouraging test report, I indulged in a temper tantrum of epic proportions. Raging, crying, cursing—silenced only by great slurps of scotch—I vented my fears and anger. The children scattered, though there was no way they could escape my shrill complaints. Except for my cacophony, the house was still, ghostlike. Later, worn out and sniveling, I lay in bed, alone, considering my dismal future. Ken, our oldest son, slipped quietly into the unlit room, sat next to the bed, and reached for my hand. "Mother, I just want you to know that we love you. Love you the way you are. We'll understand if you refuse to take treatment. It's your choice. And we want you to make it. We'll accept your decision because we love you." And he left. I lay there, tears streaming down my cheeks. Having been allowed to die, I wanted desperately to live.

Journal Excerpt—April, 1975

The greatest gift my family has given me is that they have made me feel successful. Each child—Cathy, Rob, and Ken—has reacted to this crisis in the most mature way—each differently as they are each different—but competently, quietly, and I guess most importantly, securely. If only I can live the rest of my life on my terms I will feel that they were left with a heritage of the best I could give. And the fact that they accepted what I gave is what gives me a real inner peace.

Because we hid nothing from them, Jack and I didn't have to talk secretly. When I had tests and was anxious about the results, I could slam doors and curse my existence and the children knew why I was angry. But there were other, far-reaching results of our decision to tell the truth. When Cathy went for professional help in picking a college, the counselor asked her how she felt about the fact that her mother was dying. She was able to come home, tell me what happened, express her anger, and refuse to go back. She and we picked her college without that insensitive bungler. When Rob asked a former employer to write a recommendation for a new job, he was shocked to find that the man wrote that he (Rob) was suffering over his mother's terminal illness. Rob's feelings, when he told me about it, were that the man was uninformed about me and ill-informed about him. He too was angry. But we discussed how other people seem to transfer their own preconceptions. We could talk because we were honest.

All parents want their children to grow up with no unhappiness, no misfortune, no hurt. But in our home, my illness gave us a chance to stretch relationships. To put our lives into perspective and to recognize priorities.

Long after the cancer spread to my neck, I was aware that Dann and I had never discussed the metastasis. We spoke around it. "How are you?" "I'm fine." And I puzzled over it. It was often hard for me to remember that he did care, that he did love me. I wanted so badly to talk to him, to tell him what I was thinking. One day he called and asked me to have lunch with him. I had recently finished my sessions with the psychiatrist and was beginning to stumble back into a state of mental health. But Dann knew none of that.

Having to call a psychiatrist had been a bitter defeat. It made me feel very inadequate. I had thought myself strong, stable, surrounded with loving interest, and I was ashamed that I needed professional help. But afterward, after only two months of therapy, I was grateful. For the psychiatrist showed me how to better use the relationships I already had. He reminded me that we are only human—not superhuman. And that while we are limited in our own strengths, we can use each other's strengths. Giving is important. Taking is important too.

I had never told Dann of my destructive state of mind. After all, we tried to make our visits a happy time. When we met for lunch, he posed his familiar, "How are you?" And this time, I told him the truth. In detail. I told him of the months of unreality, of fear and self-hate. I told him of my loneliness and need and shame. And I told him of the help I'd received from the psychiatrist. And from Norman Cousins.

Dann told me, later, he was so shocked that he had to hold himself on his chair. He had had no intimation I was anything but fine. But I have never regretted the spasm of self-indulgence I inflicted on him that day. It changed our attitudes about each other. So, late but not too late, we shared our lives. Because I was learning to deal with reality rather than what I or others wished reality to be.

Betty was experiencing her own torment as a result of my metastasis. Her predicament was, in many ways, harder than waking up to find that you have cancer. She lived with a great "what if?"—a terrifying "when?" Her sorrow for me wrestled with a gnawing concern for herself. She faced a vicious ritual of self-examination, professional checkups, acceptance of the possibilities, and the denial necessary to normalize her roles of working woman, wife, and mother.

For so long, I had used my family and friends as a shield—to protect me, by their attendance and attention, from my fears. But now I found that I was gaining control again. As I learned to verbalize my doubts, they became less awesome, more acceptable. Confrontation made them an ordinary part of my life. I could now deal with the fears the rest of my family and friends had for me and for themselves. And finally, I could be alone.

Journal Excerpt—January, 1977

I was thinking tonight of how surrounded I am by loving, caring, and apprehension. I got angry and couldn't even understand why I was angry. But then I understood that here I am—in a box—and I must operate within those parameters. Everyone, well or ill, has somewhat the same experience, I'm sure. But mine has been so dramatic and I'm just becoming aware of the problems. My first reaction is to leave—go away—but I'm sure I can adjust. It is very akin to being smothered. Maybe if the cancer will stay in abeyance for a while I can be allowed a little breathing room. It is not the routine of my life I long to escape, but the dimensions I would love to break through.

I had learned I couldn't rely only on other people for my strength. Suddenly, all the support, all the tenacity, all the love that poured toward me was inadequate. I could use it. I could depend on it, even enjoy it. But the toughness I wanted had to come from me. From inside. It was a period of learning to depend on myself, rather than drawing sustenance from others.

I could now say to my mother, "Yes. I am sick. Don't wish my illness on yourself. I can handle it. You don't have to protect me. I am not only your daughter any more. I am me. I have my own family. You cannot live for me. Stop trying. But keep loving me."

And so we all changed. Which made relationships change. It was as if we were meeting for the first time. And we needed time to get to know and feel comfortable with each other again.

Jack and I found the time to discuss and plan our lives and our deaths. Unfortunately, our culture makes death a taboo subject—so unpleasant it must be avoided. But, having come face to face with the reality of death, I needed to verbalize how I wanted to die. I told Jack how I felt about funeral homes and burial and cremation. I told him what poetry I loved and he promised to make it a part of whatever funeral service there might be. He talked about his preferences, too, and I was exhilarated by having the subject out in the open. Now I could put it behind me. Again, I silently thanked the psychiatrist for teaching me to say what I was thinking.

Faced with the vast implications that cancer provoked, I had lost my sense of perspective. Psychiatric help allowed me to see myself more sympathetically and more honestly. Playing a false role is a tremendous energy drain and I had diverted all of my vitality in the wrong directions. Once I faced my weaknesses, I could resume my strengths. I thought I knew myself when I was thirty-seven. I think I know myself today. I am not the same person.

Journal Excerpt—May, 1979

I was thirty-seven when it all started. Nine years later the conditions of my life have changed drastically. The children are grown. Jack is well established in his work, in the community, in his friendships. *I am thinking of the future differently. I'm willing to let happen what will happen. I have worked hard to get inside my head and I have learned to work toward what I really feel. I no longer need epitaphs that note my heroic nature.*

It is nine years since I found the lump. And I wonder at the changes in all of us—our relationships with each other and to our world. What differences would there be if it hadn't happened? Are we better or worse? Or perhaps the same? That couldn't be so, could it? No way! We are changed. And it is good.

Tony

When Lucy tells us of the problems she encountered in dealing with her family, we can empathize with her. The success or failure of her relationships is determined by many factors, but ultimately it is most influenced by the relationships that existed prior to the onset of her illness. And her life will be heavily affected by the support, or lack of it, of her family and close friends.

The relationship of the patient and family with the physician and surgeon is quite different but has, in my experience, followed strikingly constant patterns.

The initial instinct of almost every family in dealing with the patient who has cancer is to keep the diagnosis from the patient. The regularity of this request is extraordinary, and is equaled only by the futility and unfairness of it. It is unfair to everyone: patient, physician, and family.

A TIME FOR TRUTH

From a purely practical point of view, asking the physician to withhold the truth places him in an impossible situation, because he cannot explain the need for further diagnostic studies, possible radiation and chemotherapy, and the life-long follow-up in terms of the allegedly benign disease. In cases where mastectomy is the treatment, the truth is apparent to the patient immediately. But even in those cases, families urge us not to tell the patient the degree of spread: again, an impossible situation to reconcile with the follow-up treatment.

From another, practical point of view, asking a doctor to withhold the truth is asking him to jeopardize his whole rapport with the patient—for if he lies once and is caught at it, he may never again regain the trust and confidence that is so hard to win in this emotionally loaded setting. I have had the awful experience of having a patient who was about to undergo biopsy of a suspicious breast lump say to me just before surgery, "I know I won't be able to believe you, whatever you tell me, so I'm not going to ask you anything." This came after several hours of explaining in detail *all* options available, possible results and stages; this from a lady who read three large volumes on breast cancer prior to her biopsy! My only recourse was to tell her I would give her a preoperative key to the answers and she would not *need* to ask me. This patient was prepared for a wide local excision, axillary dissection, and radiation as primary therapy if the biopsy proved malignant.

The key was:

1. biopsy scar only (no axillary incision)
   no radiation
   no chemotherapy
   few postoperative visits and return to original referring doctor

   means: benign

2. biopsy scar
   axillary scar with suction drain
   radiation to breast postoperatively
   no chemotherapy
   lifelong follow-up by me

   means: cancer, no spread to axillary nodes, greater than 90 percent
          cure rate

3. biopsy scar
   axillary scar-suction drain
   postop radiation to breast
   postop chemotherapy
   lifelong follow-up by me *and* oncologist

   means: cancer, spread to nodes and possibly beyond, cure rate
          about 50 percent

This *barely* satisfied her doubts, and finally I promised her that I would show her the pathology report in the chart (talk about skeptics!).

Result: benign disease
          trusting, happy, and informed patient.

Start all over with the next patient to establish that trust again.

Now, why would I ever want to jeopardize that important relationship because someone in the family has this vague and ill-conceived idea that the patient is not strong enough to deal with the reality of having cancer? With the possible exception of the very senile or mentally incompetent patient, there is absolutely no reason or justification for withholding the truth.

These are the arguments that come from attitudes and convictions as a result of treating a large population of cancer patients. The legal side of the question is still more compelling: Simply stated, in almost every state, the patient has legal access to all his or her records, x-rays, and test results. We have no legal right to refuse them to the patient. In fact, in most places there is nothing to stop the patient from reading her own chart, despite the myth that has been perpetuated that the chart is some inviolable "for your eyes only — burn after reading — top secret" document. So as a practical matter we have no legal right to withhold the truth, in the same way that we have no *moral* right.

What is best for the patient? Ultimately the patient must decide. I can try to educate her and help make her decision and her consent informed. And naturally my personal views will be reflected in that advice. But the final choice as to treatment (or refusal of treatment) must lie with the patient; and that decision cannot be made if the patient has been lied to.

Another factor enters the picture here. Whether the patient survives the cancer to live a normal life or succumbs to the disease in a few months, the remaining period of time is made easiest and most natural if she and her family can talk about it openly.

A CONSPIRACY OF SILENCE

I knew a family in which the husband developed two simul-taneous cancers which would ultimately kill him within 18 months. His family insisted he not be told of the second cancer (he knew of the first). Husband and wife, children, and physician never mentioned the second and more lethal cancer for the whole 18 months. Treatment (chemotherapy) was masked under various guises, the man deteriorated piti-ably in the last months, yet no one spoke of the disease. Here was a highly intelligent man dying of cancer and he had no one to talk to. And here was a family in pain beyond bearing and unable to express it. And for what? We cannot delude ourselves into believing that he did not know all along. So there was this conspiracy of silence—a conspiracy which was, in fact, entered into mutely by the patient, for he partici-pated in this charade by never forcing the discussion. The intent of protecting him from the bad news failed and the intent of making his end easier failed, all because he had no one to talk to—he was in solitary confinement for the crime of having cancer and a family that loved him too much to hurt him. In the end his road through hell was indeed paved with good intentions.

ONE DAY AT A TIME

I have never had a cancer patient who did not suffer some depression at the discovery of his or her disease. And there is always the shadow of the Damoclean sword that follows such patients for at least five years and, in the case of breast cancer, for fifteen or twenty years. But they *all* recover from this reality with proper support, whether that support is from physician, family, friends, or even a psychiatrist. The sword becomes less visible and life goes on, simply because life can *only* go on, unless you prefer to sit in bed and wait for the end—for most people that is just boring.

It reminds me very much of a visit I made to a friend who

had just been married in Saigon in 1973. The U.S. troops had all been withdrawn from Vietnam earlier that year, but Saigon had not yet fallen to the forces of the North. When I first landed at Thansanut airport I was intensely aware of being in a country at war—of weapons, of an enemy nearby, and the reality of the possibility of death. But in hours, and certainly within a few days, the mind ignores those things, the eternal optimism of the human mind asserts itself, and soon life resumes. You go to restaurants, transact business, even drive to the beach on a Sunday despite the fact that much of the route is nominally secured by the Vietcong. Why? Because life does go on and we are all optimists deep down when it comes to survival. And even when the shelling can be heard a few kilometers outside the city, instinct says, "Not *me*. I'm safe. I'm alive. I will survive." We are all going to die—the fact is undeniable—but at the same time the fact is made tolerable only because we do not know exactly when. The patient with metastatic cancer has a better idea of *about* when, but still does not know exactly. And it is precisely that uncertainty that makes such a fate livable. If we knew the date of our death, life would be unbearable. Ignorance of this *is* bliss. I rigidly refuse to give expected survivals to families or patients for the very real reason that I do not know. Once you have given the "time," you have pronounced sentence. The patient himself can only guess, but when the guess comes from the doctor it has a certain legitimacy.

Lucy's father, in fact, was told by his doctor that he had six months to live. After his death a family member found that date circled by him on a calendar. What a cruel thing to do to him—albeit with the best of intentions.

Probably one of the most hopeless and rapidly progressive cancers is that of the pancreas. Usual survivals range from three to six months. But I have seen patients go two years! It would be terribly unfair to "sentence" that patient to six months and have him outlive that prediction, believing each day to be his last. The *quality* of his survival would then be very poor.

At this point it would be well to dispense with what I feel is a much overblown topic: euthanasia. The press and the courts have made a great deal of the question of the patient's right to die, with or without outside help. I will make no arguments for or against euthanasia, for adequate discussion would fill an entire book and is not appropriate here. We are concerned with the problems of *living* with cancer, not dying from it. My experience and that of my colleagues suggests that life is incredibly precious to most patients. It seems to revolve about the realization that we all will be dead for a very long time and so life remains very precious. Patients I have known, even those in great distress, will take whatever time we can give them; the desire to escape this life even a day earlier is by far the exception rather than the rule.

DENIAL – SHUTTING OUT THE LIGHT

Another denial of our fallibility is the instinct to spend our time enjoying the victories of surgery and avoiding our failures. It is so easy to spend time on rounds chatting with the patient recovering from having his gallbladder removed. He came in sick, had his surgery, and will soon be going home well. He is happy, the family is happy, and you enjoy the victory at hand.

But then how very hard it is to stay and spend time with the terminal or incurable patient, for he is there confronting you with your feet of clay. And yet it is this patient who needs your time, your ear, and your understanding the most. That patient who was relieved of his gallbladder is going to go home and resume his life whether or not you say a single kind word — it is the incurable patient who really needs what little you have left with which to comfort him.

Which brings us finally to the mechanisms of "denial." What if the patient does not want to know? What if he just does not want to hear it? We do run into this, though not really very often. It amazes me how consistently the sequence evolves in these patients. The patient is usually in the hospital for a biopsy or exploration. The possibility of cancer (among other things) is generally anticipated preoperatively and the options discussed with the patient. At surgery, cancer is found and treated by whatever means. The family is met in the waiting room and told all the details. The family grieves together, while the patient is still asleep in the recovery room. The variation comes when the patient is fully awake and is seen by the surgeon for the first visit after the operation. Something different occurs. One might expect to hear the following conversation:

"Was it cancer?"
"Yes."
"Did you get it all?"
"I think so."
"What now?" (etc.)

In reality, one is more likely to hear:

"Hi."
"How do you feel?"
"Sore."
"That will get better each day. Hungry?"
"Not really."

Denial — the patient has just *not* said something very important. He did not ask about cancer. In other words, he *has* said, "I do not want to know. I realize that it might have been cancer because we talked about it before surgery, but if I do not hear it from your lips, then maybe it is not so."

Handling this patient is somewhat more complicated. My own preference is to play the game by his rules. Just as he is entitled to the full truth if he wishes it, I also believe he is allowed to deny the truth, at least for a while. Later, if he broaches the subject again, I will try to make a gentle transition to the truth and ultimately I like to discuss it with both the family and patient present, so that there is less opportunity for them to confuse what they heard. People are very excitable at times of illness and it is very common to finish a detailed explanation and realize they have not registered a single word. It is generally best to go over it again at a different time or several times.

Patients are not the only ones susceptible to denial. Doctors do it, too, because they are, like the patient, human and subject to human frailties. These frailties reside in all of us, despite the patient's desire for *his* doctor to be perfect.

Our denial takes a different form. We do not have the luxury of closing our eyes to a diagnosis, but we tend to close them to our failures or our impotence.

My associate and I perform a large number of major operations each year on many critically ill patients. Once we speculated on how many of those died postoperatively. I guessed three or four; he thought six or seven. When we looked at the actual figure it was thirteen for that year. We had absolutely denied failure, even when the majority of those patients had disease which was beyond cure by any measure. Why should patients deny any less when their own lives are at stake?

The advances in modern medical technology are staggering; today we are routinely able to save patients who only five years ago routinely died. Denial merely reflects our frustration at our impotence in defeating certain diseases.

Before the advent of antibiotics, physicians must have suffered the same frustration at their helplessness in treating infectious diseases as we are faced with now in treating some forms of cancer. Recognition of the realities of life and death do not, however, diminish the frustration, and so we, too, deny.

Patient denial can also be useful. It helps some patients avoid an ugly truth, at least temporarily. However, long-term absolute denial is extremely hard on everyone and fortunately is relatively uncommon in my experience. Most patients merely require gentle transition to the truth over a period of days or weeks — occasionally months.

In the long run, the truth serves everyone best—patient, doctor, and family all benefit—and attempts to withhold the real facts invariably backfire. Gentleness and tact are essential, but in the last analysis, by every standard, the patient has the right to know.

7

Learning About Cancer

Lucy

The secret of cancer is as subtle as the secret of life itself.
— Isaac Asimov —
Intelligent Man's Guide
to Science — Vol. II

Before I had breast cancer I seldom examined my own breasts. Bombarded by television, radio, and printed matter advising us of cancer's danger signals, I still chose to ignore the simple exercise of regularly examining my own breasts. Yet, I was the one who found the lump, by chance, in the shower, New Year's Eve ten years ago. I knew, when I felt it, that it was alien, that it didn't belong to me. I knew because I was instinctively aware of my own body. How much sooner would I have detected it if I had checked myself frequently? Would it have made a difference in the course of my disease? I try not to dwell on those questions. That time is past. Guilt is destructive, and I want to concentrate on now and tomorrow. Now and tomorrow is teaching my daughter to examine her breasts.

When I had the mastectomy, I knew very little about breast cancer. I had watched my mother and my aunt survive the same operation and have no recurrence. Their subsequent good health had lulled me. Breast cancer had meant disfigurement — not metastasis, not debilitation, not death. But my cancer was different from theirs. I found myself bogged down in ignorance, dealing with mystery, fighting for direction. Had I educated myself about breast cancer before I had breast cancer, would the course of my treatment have been different? That, too, is an empty question. What has happened is done. Guilt is arrogant. Instead, I talk to my daughter and encourage her to learn what I've discovered.

After I recovered from the mastectomy, I wanted information. I wanted to know about my disease and to understand my treatment. I wanted to anticipate my future. The quickest, easiest, most available source of information was my doctors. But doctors often do not trust their patients' ability to understand the complexities and enigmas of cancer. My surgeon was afraid that too much knowledge would frighten me. He was highly skilled and totally dedicated. Yet he was nervous and fidgety when I questioned him. The radiologist was gracious with his time, but he admitted he did not like to discuss "the hairy details that might be frightening." He wanted to be open and honest, yet "hopefully reassuring." For me, however, truth has no modifiers. It might be equivocal. It might be comparative. It might change. But truth is never qualified. I needed more than the doctors would give me.

I began my self-instruction with medical texts. But I soon realized they were too technical for me to unravel. Imagine, if you will, this eager, attentive, omniverous reader — me — finding herself confused, stumbling, and confounded. Even the dictionary didn't solve my dilemma. While I had problems understanding what I read, I did become familiar with the medical terminology and could then read less technical books on such topics as cell multiplication, the endocrine system, and immunological research. It was a beginning.

I read a book which one reviewer said was ". . . an incredible account of how only the author's stubbornness in demanding that she be allowed to be treated by the surgeon of her choice saved her from suffering the tortures that are so frequently and needlessly the lot of women who submit to a breast cancer operation that has been performed almost perfunctorily for fifty years." The review had intrigued me and when I went to the bookstore to buy the book, *The Invisible Worm*, by Rosamond Campion, it couldn't be found. The clerk was confused. She was certain the book was in stock — she remembered seeing it — but where? We both searched but with no luck. I left my name and asked her to phone me when it reappeared. She called a few days later to apologize. The reason the book had been difficult to locate was that, because of its title, *The Invisible Worm*, it had been shelved under "gardening." So much for cancer books with fancy titles. But the book did make me recognize, for the first time, the choices a woman has if she but realizes them. Shopping for doctors is a viable option. A radical mastectomy was not my only choice. But because I didn't consider my alternatives, didn't ask, wasn't told, that was how I was treated.

We refuse to smoke cigarettes because cigarette smoking causes lung cancer. We avoid food additives because they are carcinogenic. We fear nuclear power because excess radiation might result in leukemia. But there is no proven agent that causes breast cancer. There are studies that show that inherited factors, a high animal fat diet, or excess hormones might be causes. These studies are only in the test stage and statistics can be manipulated. Instead of depending on inconclusive, analytical data, women should be aware of the dilemma but they should also depend on their intimate knowledge of their own bodies. And know, if they do develop breast cancer, what their options are. That, indeed, they do have options.

It is very easy to find material on breast cancer. It floods the bookstores. Magazines have articles, if not weekly, then monthly. The newspapers feature personal reports, releases from medical seminars, and drug companies. Sometimes the information is erroneous. Reporters jump the gun to report "Drugs Found To Curb Breast Cancer" or headline "Spectacular Hope" for women with breast cancer. None of that has been or is true—yet it sells magazines and newspapers. We must be sophisticated enough to weed out the hyperbole. But even misinformation will give us a platform from which to question. And questioning—direct questioning—is the only way to learn.

I devoured a mélange of books: *Conquering Cancer*, by Israel; *Breast Cancer*, by Kushner; Alsop's *Stay of Execution*; Sontag's *Illness as Metaphor*. I read articles on immunotherapy, on the right to commit suicide, on the politics of the American Cancer Society. I found ideas that corresponded with mine and thoughts that stretched my imagination. And,

happily, I found Norman Cousins' "*Anatomy of an Illness.*"*
His belief, that the will to live is a curative force, was an
irresistible lure. I had always thought of cancer in terms of
conflict: invade, kill, conquer, fight, defend. Cousins spoke
of illness in terms of possibility: believe, control, share, hope,
protect. I liked that. If I chose life, I preferred to live positively, contributing to and understanding my existence. Using
myself to be at peace with myself.

The excitement provoked by Cousins' philosophy drew
me to study the practice and technique of mind control. I
speak of mind control in terms of subjective conception
rather than ruthless coercion. In my search for a personal
philosophy, I had discovered, when my father died, and when
I got sick, that I did not find comfort or peace from a God.
Rather, I was aware, curiously, that I didn't consider any
religious dogma. Consequently, I searched for what I could
believe. My moral sense was strong, but morals are abstract
and I sought a practical, tangible vehicle for my ideas.

I found me. My mind and my body. If I could think
positively, my thoughts would affect my body. I could
transfer my will to live into a physical reality.

I read *Getting Well Again*, by the Simontons. I read *And a
Time to Live*, by Cantor. And my reflections were reinforced.
The Simontons say:

> *Because cancer is such a dread disease, the minute people know
> someone has cancer, it often becomes the person's defining
> characteristic. The individual may play numerous other roles—
> parent, boss, lover—and have numerous valuable personal charac-
> teristics—intelligence, charm, a sense of humor—but from that
> moment on he or she is a "cancer patient." The person's full
> human identity is lost to his or her cancer identity. All anyone is
> aware of, often including the physician, is the physical fact of
> cancer, and all treatment is aimed at the patient as a body, not as
> a person.*
>
> *It is our central premise that an illness is not purely a physical
> problem but rather a problem of the whole person, that it in-
> cludes not only body but mind and emotions. . . . some patients*

*Published in book form by W. W. Norton & Company, New York,
1979.

who have faced cancer and have worked to influence the course
of their disease develop a psychological strength greater than they
possessed before the illness—the feeling of being "weller than
well."

That's how I feel. Weller than well.

I discovered an organization called Hospice. Hospice is
staffed by volunteers: a medical director, registered nurses,
clergymen, social workers, and lay people. They serve the
terminally ill patient who has been referred by a physician
because active curative therapy is no longer indicated. These
volunteers help the patient to live and die according to his or
her values and beliefs, and are available to that patient
twenty-four hours a day, seven days a week. They also offer
support to the patient's family, whether at home or in the
hospital. And their assistance does not cease at the time of
death—they remain available to the family throughout the
postdeath period of grief.

Happily, I wasn't qualified to be a participant in Hospice.
But I found its existence to be a comfort. And I went to
study groups which Hospice held for its volunteers. It was
another source from which I could gain information.

But of course I never forget that the reason I have been
able to learn and feel good about learning is that I have had
time. Ten years have passed since that first dismal prognosis.
It has been five years since the metastasis.

I have had time to learn more about drugs since that
period, ten years ago, when I became addicted to drugs from
the casual dispensation of prescriptions—whereupon, simply,
my pain was cured by spending a week in traction. I have had
to withdraw from a four-year addiction to Valium, prescribed
to ease the discomfort of menopause. No doctor advised me
to stop taking it—in fact, I was encouraged to continue. But
I knew it was destructive. I had learned it was entirely unnecessary. Yet it remained for me to counsel myself. So I
have been able to say to my children, "Don't tell me that
drugs are a harmless source of pleasure. I know it is not that
simple. I was there. I was addicted. And I still felt my pain.
The pain was still there, and, worse, I lost my self-control.
Don't tell me about drugs. They are an abomination."

Most first-person accounts of breast cancer have been written within the first two years of the diagnosis. And the early days and months and years are a time of mourning, of fear, of anger. I felt those emotions. The books I read described those emotions. The cancer patients whom I talk to feel those emotions. But I am ten years from the day when I learned I had breast cancer. My priorities have changed because of time. What concerned me then—whether Jack would love me, whether I could like myself, the horrifying mutilation—have faded. I remember those concerns and celebrate—because I have been so lucky. I have had time. I have had time to know that my husband loves me *and* my lop-sided body. Isn't that wonderful? I have had time to realize that a breast is hardly more than a giant sweat gland, useful only to secrete milk. Well, I have lots of sweat glands and my children are too old to suckle. The fears and offended vanity of ten years ago have been displaced by my thoughts of the more serious consequences of my disease. Instead of wasting my time weeping over my imperfect body, I live with my scars and wrap myself, not in grief and rationalizations, but in my hopes for life.

Sometimes I wonder why it took something as dramatic as breast cancer to force me to grow up. So many people mature easily, with no sudden catastrophe to mark their perceptions. But I seemed to need to know extreme pain in order to recognize pure joy.

Is it any wonder that I exult?

And I exult because I have had time.

Tony

Every breast cancer patient has an obligation to herself and her doctor to learn at least the basics of her disease process, the treatment, and the risks involved. Unfortunately, it is easier to pass this responsibility entirely on to the doctor. When a patient is ill and frightened, it is safer to assign omniscience to the doctor because it makes the patient feel safer. It removes the responsibilities which attach to decisions involving risk. However, that attitude is a cop-out. Physicians are neither infallible nor omniscient.

TO ERR IS HUMAN

Pope told us succinctly that fallibility is part of the human condition. More recently, Lewis Thomas, in his *The Medusa and the Snail*,* points out that it is this very fallibility that not only separates us from lower forms of life, but actually gives us our greatest opportunities to improve. He tells us:

> *We are at our human finest, dancing with our minds, when there are more choices than two. Sometimes there are ten, even twenty different ways to go, all but one bound to be wrong, and the richness of selection in such situations can lift us onto totally new ground. This process is called exploration and is based on human fallibility. If we had only a single center in our brains, capable of responding only when a correct decision was to be made . . . we could only stay the way we are today, stuck fast.*

But patients do not want the doctor to be fallible when it comes to treating them. They want him on that pedestal, and

*New York, Viking Press, 1974, page 39.

they are angry if they see him step down. There is a worn-out joke that used to circulate in the hospitals about a long line of people who are waiting their turn to enter heaven, when a man in a white coat, carrying a black bag and stethoscope, walks ahead of everyone and enters the pearly gates in front of the crowd. When one of the people in line protests, St. Peter quickly steps in and says, "Oh don't mind Him — that's God. He likes to play doctor every now and then."

The fact is, the vast majority of doctors do not have that godlike self-image, despite public opinion to the contrary. Indeed, they feel burdened by such implications and recognize that medicine today, despite all its sophistication and space-age technology, is still, in large part, as much art as science.

For every clear-cut, indisputable solution, there is another case in which the borders are fuzzy and judgments are very subjective. This is where the educated patient plays an important role. In problems involving several choices, the patient needs to be presented with sufficient data to participate in the decisions. Black and white is easy. Gray requires something more.

Lucy began her journey as a liberally educated medical illiterate. She asked no questions because she did not know what to ask. Naturally, she got to make no decisions. At the time of her surgery, classic Halsted radical mastectomy was still in vogue in most places, but many surgeons had already turned to modified radical mastectomy. Lumpectomy with radiation was not popular, but at least one major university center in the region where she lived was performing this type of surgery. At that time, there was no right or wrong way, any more than there is today, but there *was* a choice. Lucy did not have the basic facts to know there *was* such a choice, much less to make an intelligent decision as to which might be best for her. We are not trying to argue legal points of informed consent, but rather to emphasize that much of medicine involves choices, and the doctor should not always make those choices alone.

In school we suspected that one of the teachers graded papers by the old staircase method, so on one exam we all wrote, "Check here if you've read this far." He hadn't. However, if *you've* read this far, you are obviously interested in learning more than the fact that cancer can occur in the breast. What then are other sources available to the interested patient, or potential patient?

WARNING: INFORMATION FROM YOUR FRIENDS ON BREAST CANCER MAY BE HAZARDOUS TO YOUR HEALTH

The very first realization which every patient must make is that she is unique, her disease is unique, and her treatment and course will be unique. This may be more applicable to breast cancer than to almost any other disease. As discussed earlier, the usual five-year survivals as parameters of cure do not apply in breast cancer, as they do to other cancers, and the multiple modalities of treatment (surgery, radiation, chemotherapy, hormone manipulations, as well as variations within those modalities) make comparisons between individual patients impossible. Indeed, valid studies generally involve literally hundreds of cases followed for many years.

The only valid comparisons that can be made are from *prospective randomized control studies.* This term means that the study is set up to examine patients treated in a specific medical regimen, compared with a matched group (age, sex, degree of disease) treated by another method. The group to which the patient is assigned is selected at random, and the results of treatment are analyzed by an independent party who does not know what treatment the patient had. This is known as the *double blind* technique and assures impartiality (cynics refer to double blind studies as those in which no one knows what is going on). The ethics involved here require that all patients who volunteer be apprised of all risks and possible benefits, especially when trials require comparing one drug against a placebo (no real treatment at all). In the best of circumstances it is difficult to get sufficient volunteers to gather adequate data. The National Cancer Institute recently set up a program comparing modified radical mastectomy with lumpectomy followed by radiation. They needed 300 patients to get acceptable statistics (recall that about 110,000 women will develop breast cancer this year). After four months only 12 women volunteered, despite the fact that two very well-tried choices were being compared. Patients just do not want to give up their right to choose.

Imagine the difficulty when we need to compare several modes of surgical therapy, with and without several chemotherapeutic agents, radiation, and hormone manipulation. Add to that pre- and postmenopausal status, and you can see that the variables are legion and that good prospective controlled studies are extremely difficult to obtain, especially in breast cancer, for which five-year follow-ups are not enough; ten-, fifteen-, and twenty-year protocols are required.

So when your neighbor arrives to relate the detailed agonies of her sister's cousin's aunt, the best thing to do is to disregard every detail.

A similar caveat should apply to virtually all the media; e.g., *Time* magazine might also be hazardous to your health. Normalcy is not newsworthy, and although many of the major breakthroughs are eventually reported in the press, these reports are generally released prematurely and with little sophistication in their analysis. Medical literature is staggering in its sheer volume, and most physicians can barely keep up with the changes reported weekly or monthly in even the most narrow of specialties. It would not be unusual for a general surgeon to receive monthly editions of *The American Journal of Surgery*, *Annals of Surgery*, *Archives of Surgery*, *Surgery*, *Gynecology and Obstetrics*, and *Surgical Clinics of North America*, as well as weekly editions of *JAMA (Journal of the American Medical Association)* and the *New England Journal of Medicine*. Needless to say, careful assessment of the articles in these few journals would require more hours than exist in the day. Furthermore, despite the careful selection by the editing panels of these publications, the articles are very variable in their applicability and validity. The conclusions of different articles may be completely contradictory. My final exam in a statistics course in medical school was to analyze the figures used in a study reporting that removal of a normal appendix was associated with the later development of colon cancer. This appeared in a reputable journal and was published by sincere investigators who believed in their conclusions. However, even third-year medical students were able to see the flaws in the study once statistical analysis was applied. Lies, damned lies, and statistics.

Unfortunately, the members of the press are even less able to sift out the good from the bad in medical reporting, and their emphasis on the sensational has too often obscured the realities of clinical application. Even in today's world, where technology is expanding at a dizzying rate, changes in medicine come slowly, often after long clinical trials and years of data gathering. The press too often heralds a new breakthrough only to disappoint those who may have to wait years before the new knowledge can be applied to the public at large.

Where then *does* one go to get the story? The first step should be the selection of the doctor (or doctors, when more than one opinion is warranted). Once a relationship has been established, a competent doctor can be your primary source of information. Despite preexisting opinions regarding your particular case, it is your doctor's obligation to make you aware of all the significant choices and the various risks and benefits of each. You should not expect nor be expected to pass an exam on the pathologic anatomy of your disease, but you should expect to have sufficient information upon which to base your decisions.

An educated patient is the greatest asset to both the doctor and herself and within the limits of time and technology every effort should be made to obtain the information, whether it comes from the primary physician, the specialist, the second opinion, or specific patient-oriented literature, such as that disseminated by the American Cancer Society or medical associations. A little knowledge is indeed a dangerous thing, but nobody said we cannot try for *more* than a little knowledge.

8

Looking
Ahead

Lucy

Conceptions from the past blind us to facts which almost slap us in the face.

W. A. Halsted

Dr. Halsted, ironically, is the surgeon who, almost 100 years ago, invented the radical mastectomy. Until recently, this was the accepted procedure used to treat breast cancer. And Halsted's perceptions of how cancer spread were the justification for the radical surgery advised until recently by most surgeons — surgeons blinded by the concepts of the past.

Today, attitudes are changing. Research has "slapped us in the face," challenging the need for radical surgery in many cases. The results must be given time and further testing, but there is growing evidence that less mutilating surgery, coupled with radiation and/or chemotherapy, is just as effective as the Halsted mastectomy.

Most doctors now agree that a two-stage procedure is the proper method to adopt in confronting possible breast cancer surgery. When I had my mastectomy, I was informed that a biopsy would be performed, and if the pathology proved negative, or benign, I would be returned to my hospital room. If a malignancy were found, the radical surgery would take place immediately. I signed papers agreeing to such steps. I had never heard the term *two-stage procedure*. And if I had, I don't know if I could have dealt with it because I was so frightened. Part of my fear was of cancer. But my fear was caused, too, by ignorance. If I had known more about breast cancer before I had breast cancer, I might have dealt more competently with the realities and possibilities.

I often ask myself the question, "Is the horror of breast cancer caused by the fear of cancer and possible death? Or is it the terror of losing a breast, living maimed?" And I realize the two fears are entwined unalterably at first; that the invasion of the body by the knife is as abhorrent as the invasion of the body by disease. However, with time, perspective must displace some of the anguish induced by the amputation.

Breast cancer could be a very private affair. No one would have to know. Oh, people learned I had cancer and they knew that I had lost a breast. But if I had chosen not to speak further of it, they would have forgotten. There is nothing about me that screams "breast cancer." I wear pretty clothes. I play tennis and ride horseback and hike and swim. I could even wear a slinky, skimpy bathing suit (if the rest of my body were slinky and skimpy), and no one would realize I have only one breast. If I had bone cancer and had lost a leg, it would be obvious I was sick. Or if part of my jaw had been removed, people would be ever aware. A breast is dispensable. The loss of one can be hidden. Cancer — the disease cancer — is what must concern me.

Because of the new techniques available, women must accept the responsibility of knowing about breast cancer treatment, so that, if the circumstance arises, they will be able to discuss the alternative treatments suggested by their doctors. We must recognize that surgeons are performing lumpectomies and subsequent radiation implants. We must know which drugs are available and the manifestations of those drugs when they are intermingled. We should understand, before it happens, what reactions are possible, whether we can accept them, and what our choices might be.

We try to avoid unpleasantness. The radiologist once accused me of "paying the toll before I got to the bridge." But if we wait until disease threatens or metastasis occurs, our fears often prohibit an objective examination of our options. And each day new drugs are being used, new procedures are replacing old, lives are lengthened. We are obligated to be cognizant of it all. Ultimately, we must be responsible for ourselves.

When a friend had her mastectomy, she was urged to have her breast reconstructed. The procedure is major surgery and, while not for everyone, it has become more popular in the last five years. The American Cancer Society now offers a booklet entitled *Facts Every Woman Should Know About Breast Reconstruction.*

My friend refused the operation for two reasons. For one thing, reconstructive surgery is not without risk. Those risks include infection, tampering with the success of cancer treatment, and the sloughing off or hardening of the implant. She found the risks too great. She also felt that she would be fooling herself. She was shown pictures of reconstructed breasts. They weren't pretty. Rather, the choice seemed to be whether she wanted to wear her prosthesis under or on top of her skin. She examined her choices and made her decision.

The decision must be a personal one. Age and circumstance will be a determinant. But the thought occurs to me that the selling of reconstructive surgery is an insidious reminder of our cultural breast worship. The operation says specifically, "I will make you as you were before. You will be a woman again." The threat of breast cancer must be realized as a threat to life — not a threat to femininity. We must be honest. And we must realize priorities.

For me, the way to live well with cancer is to know all I can know — about the disease, about myself. And by knowing, to force the illness to fit the way I choose to live. I can insist that the doctors answer my questions because my questions are informed, based on fact. I keep a notebook with every scrap of information — every article I read, every rumor I hear, every doubt and every fear and every hope.

The way for me to live well with cancer is to be honest. To talk about how I feel and what I feel. To allow myself to be frightened and despair. To share with Jack the realities of my threatened existence.

And the way to live well with cancer is to want to live. To know that there are things I have to do. That I am needed. That there is unknown joy on the threshold. To know that I can control my life — have controlled it — will control it.

But Robinson Jeffers says it so well in "The Answer":

Then what is the answer? — Not to be deluded by dreams,
To know that great civilizations have broken down into violence,
and their tyrants come, many times before.

*When open violence appears, to avoid it with honor or choose
    the least ugly faction; these evils are essential.*
*To keep one's own integrity, be merciful and uncorrupted
    and not wish for evil; and not be duped*
*By dreams of universal justice or happiness. These dreams will
    not be fulfilled.*
*To know this, and know that however ugly the parts appear
    the whole remains beautiful. A severed hand*
*Is an ugly thing, and man dissevered from the earth and stars
    and his history . . . for contemplation or in fact . . .*
*Often appears atrociously ugly. Integrity is wholeness,
    the greatest beauty is*
*Organic wholeness, the wholeness of life and things, the
    divine beauty*
of the universe. Love that, not man
*Apart from that, or else you will share man's pitiful confusions,
    or drown in despair when his days darken.*

Copyright 1937 and renewed 1965 by
Donnan Jeffers and Garth Jeffers.
Reprinted from
The Selected Poetry of Robinson Jeffers,
by Robinson Jeffers,
by permission of Random House, Inc.

I go to my room and stand before the mirror. The health, joy, expectancy reflect back on me, and I celebrate. There has been time — ten years.

I have survived — ten years.

I want more.

Tony

Although I may have been hard on the media for their premature release of information, I should also point out that, conversely, we in medicine tend to move very slowly and cautiously when it comes to change. Indeed, some of our most spectacular advances have been delayed for long periods of time because of this cautiousness, and other advances sat there screaming to be discovered while we ignored them. Alexander Fleming discovered that penicillium mold inhibited bacterial growth on some of his laboratory cultures (someone's sloppy lab technique allowed the cultures to be contaminated by the penicillium mold). He even suggested that this "antibiosis" might be a useful way to treat bacterial infection. Yet it was fully fifteen years before Florey first applied this to the treatment of human infection in soldiers during World War II. On the other hand, we must not lose sight of the fact that ill-advised enthusiasm has also taken its toll — witness the tragedy of the thalidomide debacle.

So a fine line exists between overzealous experimentation and overcautious conservatism in the advance of medicine, and it is hard to be critical of the physician who is reluctant to abandon an old friend, be it operation or drug therapy, that may have served his patients well for many years. Polonius had a point when he said, "The friends thou hast, and their adoption tried, grapple them unto thy soul with hoops of steel; but do not dull thy palm with entertainment of each new-hatched, unfledg'd comrade."

THROUGH THE LOOKING GLASS

Halsted's radical mastectomy was a courageous operation in its day, and it has served the cause well for generation after generation. The change to modified radical mastectomy, which really only involved the sparing of the pectoralis major muscle, was many years in gaining acceptance despite the fact that it violated virtually no rules of tumor asepsis or radical surgery. Now we are in a time when, in a few areas, surgeons are testing the lumpectomy and radiation technique in an attempt to do less mutilating surgery while still achieving comparable cure rates. It may not be penicillin, but neither, we hope, will it be thalidomide. In any event, while we have pretty much seen the end of the classic radical mastectomy, the lumpectomy and radiation technique is still a long way from supplanting the modified radical mastectomy as the standard against which all new therapy must be compared. However, we *are* far enough along this road to expect that women should be given the facts and allowed a voice in this decision. As noted previously, the National Cancer Institute recently began a prospective study to compare these two techniques for which a minimum of 300 patient volunteers are needed to assure sound statistical comparison. Although these patients would be randomized as concerns treatment used, between September, 1979, and January, 1980, only *twelve* volunteers were obtained. Clearly, the patients themselves are as conservative as the doctors when it comes to their own individual fates.

The changeover is not easy. When my partner and I decided to reverse our stand and suggest lumpectomy and radiation to our patients instead of mastectomy, we wondered how patients who had just undergone mastectomy would feel when they learned of the change. How difficult would it be to have had the last mastectomy? Inwardly we hoped it would not come up. We were wrong.

I walked into the office one afternoon and noticed two patients in animated conversation in the waiting room. I got a very uneasy feeling when I realized that one of the last mastectomy patients was talking to our first lumpectomy patient—both back for a follow-up visit.

Later I had to go in and examine the patient who had had the mastectomy. She sat with her eyes brimming, and though my heart sank, she said, "Isn't it wonderful that you won't have to do this operation anymore?" It is wonderful to encounter such a generous and intelligent person.

It *is* difficult to change, and it will continue to be, but we cannot be forced to relive the past just to spare feelings once we believe the new treatment is better. In this case it will be a painful transition, but a necessary one if present results continue to hold up.

Penicillin was hailed as the "magic bullet," because it was lethal to bacteria while virtually nontoxic to human cells. Thus far no "magic bullet" has been found for breast cancer. Chemotherapeutic agents and radiation are all damaging to healthy cells as well as to cancer, and only the differential toxicity allows us to use them — and then only with the greatest of care. Someday such a "magic bullet" may make all the present modes of treatment archaic, but for the moment none is on the horizon.

MENS SANA IN CORPORE SANO

Somewhat closer on our horizon is an area known as mind control, which is still in its infancy. These techniques employ methods which are difficult to assess and do not easily lend themselves to objective evaluation.

There has, for a long time, been the impression that one's own attitude and determination (or lack of it) may play a vital role in the battle against cancer as well as several other illnesses, and doctors everywhere are impressed with the effect upon illness of the patient's will to survive. We have all seen patients who, despite the failure of traditional therapy, refuse to be defeated, as well as those who just give up and succumb for no apparent reason. About six years ago I operated on an elderly man with cancer of the colon. At surgery he was found to have an operable tumor in his colon and also a solitary metastasis in his liver. The decision was made to remove both the primary cancer in his colon and the portion of his liver with the metastasis — in spite of the statistical likelihood that more microscopic spread had already occurred in his liver. He survived the surgery and lived longer than the usual five-year time period free of disease. He was cured of his colon cancer despite the spread to the liver. In his sixth year, he developed a *new* primary cancer in his pancreas — an unusually lethal tumor. We elected to do a very radical operation despite the high risk and poor cure rate for this form of cancer. He survived this enormous operation and the many complications usually associated with it. But his wife kept telling me that the fight had gone out of him, that he seemed to have lost the will to live. The appearance of this second cancer was more than he could bear after the long struggle with his first cancer. Nearly two months later he was dead. His wounds were healed. His normal functions were restored, yet he languished in bed, ate only when forced to, and smiled politely and knowingly to our entreaties to eat. He just ran out of steam and the will to fight anymore, and so he died, ostensibly free of cancer. No earth-shaking conclusions should be drawn from this, but the story is not unusual. There is some hard to define factor involved in recovering from illness, and it still eludes precise scientific medicine. Dr. O. Carl Simonton and Stephanie Simonton have devoted a great deal of time and study to this phenomenon, and their book, *Getting Well Again*, details many of these cases, both successful and unsuccessful.

Mind control is being used in several centers on two levels: on the one hand, mind control as a form of self-hypnosis has been used to eliminate the need for narcotics in the control of pain and to restore patients to a full and useful life even when the tumor continues to progress.

On a second and more difficult to explain level, patients are trained to control their vital functions at a cellular level to enhance their tumor-fighting capabilities. Some theorize an ability to marshal resources which may actually strengthen their defenses and even cause tumor regression. Conclusive studies on this subject are still far off in the distance, but we do know that there is some host–tumor relationship that permits some cancers to kill in some months or even weeks, while the same tumor in a similar stage may be staved off for years or even regress to the point of apparent cure. Whether this represents natural spontaneous remission of the tumor itself or host defense (or both) is not clear, but it remains an intriguing problem which will bear close watching in the years to come.

WANTED: AN OUNCE OF PREVENTION

The most desirable state of affairs would be the discovery of a way to prevent breast cancer rather than just to treat it. Unfortunately, no anticancer vaccine exists. Except for decreasing the dietary intake of animal fats and choosing your parents carefully, we have no promising suggestions to stop the development of cancer in the breast.

VARIATIONS ON PROPHYLACTIC MASTECTOMY

The most direct but least desirable approach to preventing cancer would be the removal of the breast in the high-risk patient. It is not unlike removing a normal appendix to prevent later appendicitis. But in the case of mastectomy, the implications are far more serious.

Though some family histories are so strong as to warrant consideration of prophylactic simple mastectomies (removal of all breast tissue, skin, and nipples), few doctors would advise it, and fewer women would choose that option. Most would choose to be carefully examined at frequent intervals and to deal with the cancer when and if it appeared.

A compromise is subcutaneous mastectomy, in which the breast tissue is removed, but skin and nipples are left in place, much like scooping out the pulp of a melon without disturbing the rind. The breast is often rebuilt later with synthetic implants, usually after a delay of 8 to 12 months. This delay is to avoid damage to the skin which can be injured if implants are done immediately. The cosmetics of subcutaneous mastectomy may leave something to be desired, but it certainly surpasses mastectomy. Some breast tissue, and especially that of the ducts in the nipple, remains in place after subcutaneous mastectomy so that the protection is theoretically less than that of mastectomy. Insufficient numbers of cases have been done for us to know with certainty if there is a true difference between these two techniques.

BEING WHOLE AGAIN

There are several reconstruction techniques used after mastectomy. The exact details vary depending upon whether there has been a prophylactic simple mastectomy, a modified radical mastectomy, or a classic Halsted radical mastectomy with the removal of the pectoralis major muscle. Obviously, the latter will require more extensive surgery.

While details of technique are beyond the scope of this book, most operations require several stages to mobilize skin flaps from the abdomen or chest and rearrangement of subcutaneous tissue with grafts from the vulva to reconstruct a nipple.

For most women, even a close approximation of normal breast appearance is worthwhile. But the reality is that even in the hands of the most experienced plastic surgeon, there will be scarring and some discrepancy between the normal breast and the reconstructed breast. The decision to undergo the multiple operations which are usually involved, the expense, and the possible risks is a purely individual one and each woman must make that decision based on myriads of personal factors. However, she should make a careful inquiry into the surgery involved and a survey of photographs of the results of the surgeon's prior cases. The option to rebuild is reasonable, but it is not for every woman.

WAITING FOR THE MAGIC BULLET

Breast cancer, in general, is almost unique in that we have such a multitude of effective weapons at our disposal. Hopefully, surgery will play a smaller and smaller role in treatment as other modalities are advanced and refined. The combinations of surgery, radiation, chemotherapy, and hormone manipulations give us an arsenal unequaled by those available for any other tumor. The magic bullet is still many years away, as is effective prevention. Until we find one of these solutions, we must recognize that the therapeutic arsenal is indeed well supplied.

Epilogue

Almost eleven years have gone by since that New Year's Eve when Lucy first noticed a lump in her breast. Years filled with surgery, radiation, hormone ablation, scans, biopsies, more scans—fear, panic, rejoicing. Eleven years have passed since Tony felt the inadequacies inherent in trying to advise Lucy on the many possible courses of treatment. During that time he abandoned the classic radical mastectomy for the slightly more acceptable modified radical mastectomy; and now, with visible relief after a long evaluation, has adopted lumpectomy and radiation for his patients.

Lucy is ten years beyond the surgical choices, but she still wonders what lies ahead for her. The waiting and the terror at each new examination will probably never go away. But for Lucy, and all women who have had or will have breast cancer, there are good reasons for hope and reasons to never say die.

Appendixes

Appendix A

TNM CLASSIFICATION AS APPLIED TO CARCINOMA OF THE BREAST

Primary Tumor(T)

TX   Tumor cannot be assessed

TO   No evidence of primary tumor

T1S   Paget's disease of the nipple with no demonstrable tumor

T1*   Tumor 2 cm or less in greatest dimension

     T1a   No fixation to underlying pectoral fascia or muscle

     T1b   Fixation to underlying pectoral fascia and/or muscle

T2*   Tumor more than 2 cm but not more than 5 cm in its greatest dimension

     T2a   No fixation to underlying pectoral fascia and/or muscle

     T2b   Fixation to underlying pectoral fascia and/or muscle

T3*   Tumor more than 5 cm in its greatest dimension

     T3a   No fixation to underlying pectoral fascia and/or muscle

     T3b   Fixation to underlying pectoral fascia and/or muscle

T4   Tumor of any size with direct extension to chest wall or skin

     T4a   Fixation to chest wall

     T4b   Edema (including peau d'orange), ulceration of skin of breast, or satellite skin nodules confined to same breast

     T4c   Both T4a and T4b characteristics

     T4d   Inflammatory carcinoma

Nodal Involvement (N)

NX   Regional lymph nodes cannot be assessed clinically

NO   No palpable homolateral axillary nodes

N1   Movable homolateral axillary nodes

     N1a   Nodes not considered to contain growth

     N1b   Nodes considered to contain growth

From Manual for Staging of Cancer 1977. Chicago, Ill., American Joint Committee for Cancer Staging and End-Results Reporting, 1977, pp 101–104.

*Dimpling of skin, nipple retraction, or any other skin changes except those in T4b may occur in T1, T2, or T3 without the classification.

N2   Homolateral axillary nodes containing growth and fixed to one
        another or to other structures
N3   Homolateral supraclavicular or infraclavicular nodes containing
        growth or edema of arm[†]

Distant Metastasis (M)

MX   Not assessed
MO   No (known) distant metastasis
M1   Distant metastasis present; specify site

Stage Grouping

Stage I   T1a, NO or N1a
                T1b, NO or N1a, MO
Stage II   TO, N1b
                T2a, NO or N1a or N1b
                T2b, NO or N1a or N1b, MO
Stage III   Any T3, N1 or N2, MO
Stage IV   T4, any N, any M
                Any T, N3, any M
                Any T, any N, M1

[†]Homolateral internal mammary nodes considered to contain growth
are included in N3 for surgical-evaluative classification and postsurgical
treatment-pathologic classification.

How to examine your breasts

This simple 3-step procedure could save your life by finding breast cancer early when it is most curable

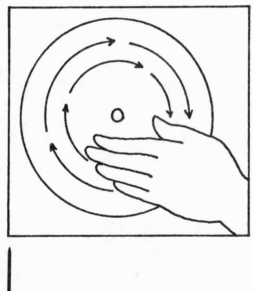

American Cancer Society

[Reproduced by permission and through the courtesy of the American Cancer Society.]

How to examine your breasts

1

In the shower:

Examine your breasts during bath or shower; hands glide easier over wet skin. Fingers flat, move gently over every part of each breast. Use right hand to examine left breast, left hand for right breast. Check for any lump, hard knot or thickening.

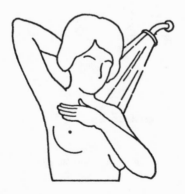

Before a mirror:

Inspect your breasts
with arms at your sides.
Next, raise your arms
high overhead. Look
for any changes in
contour of each breast,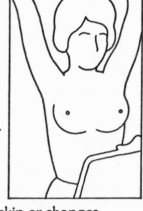
a swelling, dimpling of skin or changes
in the nipple.

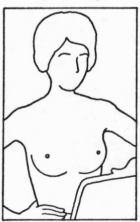 Then, rest palms on hips and press down
firmly to flex your chest
muscles. Left and right
breast will not exactly
match—few women's
breasts do.

Regular inspection
shows what is normal for
you and will give you
confidence in your
examination.

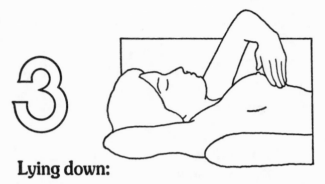

Lying down:

To examine your right breast, put a pillow or folded towel under your right shoulder. Place right hand behind your head—this distributes breast tissue more evenly on the chest. With left hand, fingers flat, press gently in small circular motions around an imaginary clock face. Begin at outermost top of your right breast for 12 o'clock, then move to 1 o'clock, and so on around the circle back to 12. A ridge of firm tissue in the lower curve of each breast is normal. Then move in an inch, toward the nipple, keep circling to examine *every part of your breast,* including nipple. This requires at least three more circles. Now slowly repeat procedure on your left breast with a pillow under your left shoulder and left hand behind head. Notice how your breast structure feels.

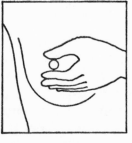

Finally, squeeze the nipple of each breast gently between thumb and index finger. Any discharge, clear or bloody, should be reported to your doctor immediately.

WHY YOU SHOULD EXAMINE YOUR BREASTS MONTHLY

Most breast cancers are first discovered by women themselves. Since breast cancers found early and treated promptly have excellent chances for cure, learning how to examine your breasts properly can help save your life. Use the simple 3-step breast self-examination (BSE) procedure shown here.

FOR THE BEST TIME TO EXAMINE YOUR BREASTS:

Follow the same procedure once a month about a week after your period, when breasts are usually not tender or swollen. After menopause, check breasts on the first day of each month. After hysterectomy, check your doctor or clinic for an appropriate time of the month. Doing BSE will give you monthly peace of mind and seeing your doctor once a year will reassure you there is nothing wrong.

WHAT YOU SHOULD DO IF YOU FIND A LUMP OR THICKENING

If a lump or dimple or discharge is discovered during BSE, it is important to see your doctor as soon as possible. Don't be frightened. Most breast lumps or changes are not cancer, but only your doctor can make the diagnosis.

Know Cancer's Warning Signals!

Change in bowel or bladder habits
A sore that does not heal
Unusual bleeding or discharge
Thickening or lump in breast or elsewhere
 Indigestion or difficulty in swallowing
Obvious change in wart or mole
Nagging cough or hoarseness

If you have a warning signal, see your doctor.

 American Cancer Society

Glossary

Adrenalectomy. Surgical removal of the adrenal glands, performed to eliminate the adrenals as a source of circulating estrogens in patients with metastatic breast cancer who have previously undergone removal of their ovaries.

Adrenal glands. Two glands situated on top of each kidney, which produce several important hormones. Their importance in breast cancer lies in their ability to produce estrogens as well.

Anaplasia. The cellular loss of distinguishing characteristics —one of the criteria of malignancy.

Aspiration. Removal of fluid by suction. Usually performed by insertion of a needle and hypodermic syringe.

Axilla. The armpit.

Axillary lymph nodes. Those lymph nodes located within the armpit which filter lymph flow from the breast. These nodes are generally the first site of regional breast cancer spread. See also **Lymph nodes: axillary levels.**

Biopsy. Removal of tissue from a living patient for examination under the microscope.

Bone survey. X-rays of the bones to locate possible spread of cancer to the bones. This is done by conventional x-rays. See also **Scans of the bone, liver, and other organs.**

Breast prosthesis. Artificial replacement part which may be worn as an external appliance (a padded bra), or a permanent surgically implanted device (silicone implant).

Butazolidin. An anti-inflammatory drug used primarily in the treatment of pain of arthritic joint disease.

Carcinoma. A form of cancer.

Chemotherapy—agents. Those used in breast cancer include

5–fluorouracil, methotrexate, cytoxan, Adriamycin, and vincristine.

Cobalt. A metallic element, one of whose radioactive isotopes is used as the source of radiation in the treatment of cancer.

Codeine. A narcotic drug used in the treatment of pain.

Cyst. A fluid filled sac.

Cystic mastitis. Generally painful fluid engorgement within cysts of the breast.

Darvon. A non-narcotic used to alleviate pain.

Electron beam. A source of radiant energy used in cancer treatment, derived from accelerating orbiting electrons by an electromagnetic field; see also **Linear accelerator.**

Endocrine system. Those glands that secrete their hormones directly into the bloodstream or lymphatic system (e.g., thyroid, adrenals, ovaries).

Estrogen. A female hormone produced primarily in the ovaries and in smaller amounts by the adrenal glands. These may stimulate the growth of preexisting breast cancer.

Estrogen-receptor protein test (ERP). Measurement of sites within a breast cancer to which estrogen may bind and accelerate tumor growth.

False negative. An x-ray or test that shows no abnormal finding even when the abnormality is present. For example, a normal mammogram in the presence of breast cancer.

False positive. An x-ray or test which appears to show an abnormal finding even when one does not actually exist.

Halsted. See **Radical mastectomy (Halsted).**

Hormone. A chemical substance produced by the glands of the body to produce a specific effect on some organ. Estrogens, for example, produce some of the cyclic changes in the uterus as well as the physical feminine characteristics of women. They may also accelerate growth of breast cancers.

Hormone manipulation. The removal or addition of hormones to the system by either surgery (e.g., removal of ovaries) or drugs (giving male hormones).

Hospice. A support organization serving the special needs of the terminally ill patient and the patient's family.

Hypophysectomy. Removal or destruction of the pituitary gland in the brain. In breast cancer it is used to stop stimulation of the adrenals and reduce estrogen production of the adrenal gland. It is a surgical alternative to removal of the adrenal glands.

Invasion. Penetration of neighboring structures by malignant tumors.

Isotope. A variant form of any element with more or less neutrons than the common form of the element. Many of these are radioactive and used as sources of radiation energy in the treatment of breast cancer (e.g., cobalt, iridium).

Lesion. Any pathological variant of normal tissue. Breast cancer is a lesion in the breast.

Linear accelerator (LINAC). An electromagnetic machine which speeds up electrons to high velocities and is used as a source of energy in treating cancer. An alternative method to, for example, radioactive cobalt as a radiation source.

Lumpectomy. Removal of a lump. Refers to the method of treatment employing the removal of the breast cancer itself as opposed to removal of the entire breast. While this term is gaining popularity, the correct medical term is "tylectomy."

Lymph nodes. Small one-half to one inch nodular collections of cells which filter secretions of the lymphatic circulation. Their importance lies in their entrapment of malignant cells and they are, therefore, sites of early cancer spread, e.g., to the nodes in the axilla from breast cancer.

Lymph nodes: axillary levels

LEVEL I—All nodes lateral to the pectoralis minor muscle.
LEVEL II—All nodes beneath the pectoralis minor muscle.
LEVEL III—All nodes medial to the pectoralis minor muscle.

Spread of cancer generally progresses from Levels I to II to III. However, prognostic differences may be better reflected by the number of positive nodes than the apparent levels.

Mammogram. X-ray of the breast, used to detect cancer.

Mastodynia. Painful breasts.

Metastasis. Spread of cancer to an anatomic site at a distance from the original cancer, e.g., breast cancer metastatic to the liver. One of the criteria of malignancy.

Modified radical mastectomy. Removal of the whole breast and axillary lymph nodes. Differs from radical mastectomy by leaving the pectoral muscles intact.

Oncologist. Medical specialist in the treatment of cancer.

Oophorectomy. Removal of the ovaries; also known as ovariectomy.

Palpable. Capable of being felt.

Palpate. To feel (with the fingers).

Partial mastectomy. Removal of only part of the breast. In cancer, the removal of the actual cancer and some amount of normal margins surrounding the cancer.

Pectoral muscle. Large fan-shaped muscle of the chest wall extending from the breastbone (sternum) to the upper arm. Its significance is its position directly beneath the breast. Its removal is part of the Halsted radical mastectomy.

Polyp. Benign growth of tissue on a stalk.

Radiation implant. Radioactive elements inserted into the body near or into the site of cancer. Used to deliver high doses of radiation to a very small area, e.g., iridium implants into the breast in breast cancer.

Rad. Unit of energy used in defining amounts of radiation.

Radiation therapy. Treatment of breast cancer with radiation energy; most commonly cobalt or electron beam in breast cancer.

Radical mastectomy (Halsted). Removal of the entire breast, pectoralis major and minor muscles, and all axillary lymph nodes.

Scans of the bone, liver, and other organs. Radioactive isotopes used to locate metastatic cancer in specific organs. Radiation doses are low and are not used for treatment of the tumors, but rather to locate them.

Seconal. A barbiturate drug used to induce sleep.

Stages of breast cancer. (See also Appendix A.)

    I—Small size, generally less than 2.5 centimeters. Negative axillary nodes. No distant spread (metastases).

    II—Small size, positive nodes. No distant spread.

    III—Large size, usually positive nodes. No distant spread.

    IV—Distant spread.

Subcutaneous mastectomy. Removal of breast tissue leaving much of the skin and nipple intact.

Tamoxifen. A drug used as an antiestrogen.

Thermography. Technique for measuring heat emission from increased blood supply to cancerous tissue.

Tumor. Any lump; may be malignant or benign.

Tylectomy. See Lumpectomy.

Valium. A tranquilizing drug used primarily to treat anxiety.

Xeromammogram. A variant using a different film than x-ray film, and a different technique resulting in clearer definition of breast anatomy and pathology.

Index

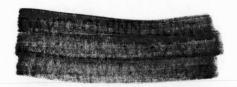